Rethinking PINK

Rethinking PINK
by Krystal Gill

XULON ELITE

Xulon Press Elite
2301 Lucien Way #415
Maitland, FL 32751
407.339.4217
www.xulonpress.com

© 2022 by Krystal Gill

All rights reserved solely by the author. The author guarantees all contents are original and do not infringe upon the legal rights of any other person or work. No part of this book may be reproduced in any form without the permission of the author. The views expressed in this book are not necessarily those of the publisher.

Due to the changing nature of the Internet, if there are any web addresses, links, or URLs included in this manuscript, these may have been altered and may no longer be accessible. The views and opinions shared in this book belong solely to the author and do not necessarily reflect those of the publisher. The publisher therefore disclaims responsibility for the views or opinions expressed within the work.

Unless otherwise indicated, Scripture quotations taken from the King James Version (KJV)–*public domain*.

Paperback ISBN-13: 978-1-6628-6080-5
Ebook ISBN-13: 978-1-6628-6081-2

Especially

For

You

Wishing you all the best
Krystal Hill
11/30/2022

In memory of my dad, who gave me more ways
to rethink pink than he knew…

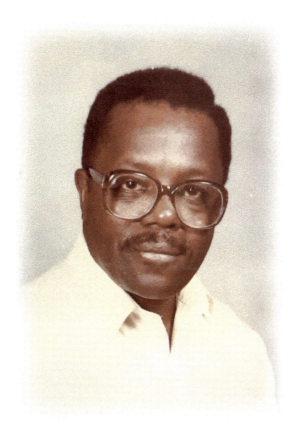

SAMUEL J. SIMMONS, JR.

ACKNOWLEDGEMENTS

I would be remiss if I did not thank the awesomely dedicated individuals who labored with me to complete my written testimony. First, I thank my professional mentor and friend Joan Burstyn, first female dean of the School of Education at Syracuse University, who has always encouraged me in my endeavors to "go for it!" Her constant reminder that she was not getting any younger at 93 has been a means of helping me to focus on my task but has also made me realize that my Heavenly Father loves me enough to keep her preserved to see me through this task. I cannot thank her enough for the readings, platforms and other means by which she has moved with me through my first publishing journey.

Much of the tone, and beauty of this book was created by my sister and best friend, Lysa Simmons of **Simmons Ink & Stitch**. Lysa has devoted many hours of listening, and creativity to my testimonial presentation and she has done it all while finding more hours in the day than I can. Her strength has truly kept me inspired to keep moving through my journey.

At first, I did not tell anyone else about my book endeavor, but spiritual strength was necessary. I thank all of my prayer partners for their love and concern for me, for the prayers known and unknown sent up on my behalf. These prayers helped me to write the toughest parts of my journey.

Yes, much can be said for the women in my life; however, it is the men in my life who have kept me grounded throughout my journey. So, I am grateful for my son for reminding me to take care of the matters of the day and my husband for never missing a moment with me through **Rethinking Pink** with his editorial assistance, personal devotion and love.

Table of Contents

Chapter 1
RETHINKING PINK 1

Chapter 2
RETHINKING REST 8

Chapter 3
RETHINKING 'WHY ME?' 18

Chapter 4
RETHINKING COMMUNITY 31

Chapter 5
RETHINKING DISABILITY 39

Chapter 6
RETHINKING FEAR 48

Chapter 7
RETHINKING PATIENCE 53

Chapter 8
RETHINKING LONELINESS 61

Chapter 9
RETHINKING PINK AGAIN 72

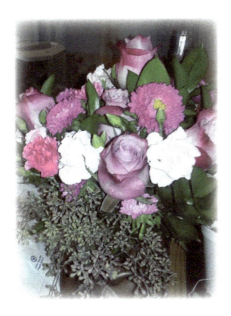

Chapter 1:

RETHINKING PINK

For he shall give his angels charge over thee, to keep thee in all thy ways.

(Psalm 91:11)

Pink, pink, you stink. Remember the childhood chant everyone seemed to know? The minute I saw one of my friends wearing pink I was quick to blurt out the chant. Even now I can hear, "Pink, pink, you stink!" echoing through my head as I recall the refrain of my early childhood days. I undoubtedly taunted my friends and others as I chanted. As far back as I can remember, I have not liked the color pink. I would not be surprised if the chant has subconsciously contributed to this notion of disdain for the color. Really. Why would anyone be comfortable wearing pink when that chant echoes through the head? Perhaps this is why we are told to be careful what we allow into our hearts because it is difficult to remove.

My clothes were not the only thing that turned me against the color pink. To me, pink was an indication of debility. I attended church where people wore flower corsages for Mother's Day. Many people wore bright red carnation corsages, some wore pink, others wore white, in honor of their mothers. I came to realize that the red corsages indicated their mothers were alive and well and pink indicated mothers were facing some infirmity. In church, one is taught to pray for that mother to get well. And for the white corsages, the unspoken announcement was that those mothers were no longer among the living. Dare I say, "Pink, pink, you stink?" Maybe not so loud but I think it stinks that death can cloud what should be what I thought was a day to express happiness. My youthful mind wondered if I would ever have to wear the pink or white flower. At the time, I could not imagine wearing any other color except red.

Did you know only real men wear pink? By the time I was in junior high school that expression was well known. Pink is the color associated with the "weaker" sex. Thanks to the social culture, pink is the rule for girls, and only girls, from birth to womanhood. Stating real men wear pink suggests the need to be granted permission to wear a desired color and then only if you are a man of strong character. Pink, pink, you stink!

My aversion to pink intensified over the years. If given a choice I almost always chose blue over pink. Blue furniture, curtains, bedspreads, bathroom fixtures. I cannot even think of anything pink in my house. Even the walls are various shades of blue paint. I have seen women's linen closets full of pink towels, sheets and blankets and I have wondered would we ever have anything in common. Pink, pink, you stink!

On September 30th, 2015, I was scheduled to have back surgery. Please know that no one wants to have back surgery. It is usually done when there is no other method of relieving the pain. I had been going to a chiropractor and had managed to have the pain in my lower back under control. But I experienced a life-changing accident December 1st, 2014. I was rethinking my decision to stay after school to catch up on grading student papers. I remember because it was my niece's birthday. I debated with myself for a while whether or not I should stay or go home, and going home won. As I went to turn off the computer on my desk, I tried to pull up the task chair and it slipped out from behind me. I fell hitting my head and the back of my neck on the windowsill behind me and my forehead on the desk in front of me. I was now on the floor too scared to move. My head was killing me. There was a nurse; two actually; and other teachers and the principal standing around me. I was embarrassed to have attracted so much attention. All I wanted was my husband. Someone called him. I was imagining him in the car driving rapidly through the streets. He must have been nervous as he got to me faster than my mind drove. I would only let him help me up. I remember my co-workers wanted me to go by ambulance, but I insisted that was not necessary, I would go to the Urgent Care Center. At Urgent Care the staff feared I had a neck fracture, so they sent me to the hospital. X-rays indicated that nothing was broken but my final diagnosis was whiplash and occipital neuralgia.

I was in constant pain. So, the doctor visits began. Even those were painful and tiresome. I stopped attending the chiropractor. This was a bad move on my part because without the routine work on my back, it became increasingly more difficult for me to get up without excruciating pain. My husband, Joseph had to assist me in the office visits that required me to lay flat on an examination table. Sometimes even with his help, the pain was intense and would take several tries before I was standing on my feet again.

Previously simple tasks were no longer simple. I could not sit or stand too long. I could not turn to the right or to the left too fast. I walked very slowly. I could not drive. I could not do basic chores; even making supper was arduous. Darkness was becoming my friend because bright light brought on migraines. I began asking myself if this was my new normal. As a woman who did not like to admit pain, I found myself fighting back the tears I was afraid would never stop if I succumbed. I needed relief. I needed a miracle.

As it turned out, I went to a church service and sat behind a friend I had not seen in a while. I remember thinking, "She's a nurse. Maybe she can lead me to a good primary care physician." After the service concluded, we did the normal things friends do: we greeted, hugged, and kissed, and then she asked, "How are you doing?" Finally, I was able to share my story, and without hesitation she offered the name of a good primary care physician (PCP). And what an awesome PCP she was! Not only did I like my new doctor, but I also loved her! Immediately I felt as though she could hear my actual complaints. It had long been obvious to me, even before my fall, that my prior PCP would dismiss my concerns and I would leave the office feeling unheard and frustrated. Even so, he had referred me to a neurologist who took an MRI, but he found it difficult to determine what was wrong and referred me to another specialist in Buffalo. But the scheduled appointment was over another three months. My new PCP had me in the hands of an outstanding neurologist in less than a week. I never thought I would be so excited to go to a doctor, but I was, and I thanked God for getting things rolling. I was getting tired of the pain.

After tests were taken, there was good news and bad news according to the neurologist. The good news: Because I had drop foot—a condition in which I cannot pick up my foot when I walk—I was tested for multiple sclerosis. I did not have MS as suspected. Truly that was good news. The bad news: I had compression of the spine which would lead to paralysis if I refused surgery. I do not think I heard this because what I did hear was that there was a greater possibility that I would be able to walk without the leg brace I was presently wearing to aid the drop foot that had worsened over the years. How I longed to be able to walk in the beautiful neighborhood where God had allowed us to find a home. How much more I longed to hang my brace on the "evidence of healing" wall at church.

I remember thinking, "Doctor, you've got it all wrong. There is no bad news here. It's all good!" Well almost all good. The neurologist sent me to see the surgeon who was ready to perform surgery immediately after viewing my MRI pictures. I told him that I was scared but before he could say "I know", I heard the Spirit say. "No you're not." Somehow, this calmed me. A feeling of peace was present, and I repented because I knew I was in the hands of God. From then on, I heard myself thanking God for the wonder of being able to walk again. As odd as it may seem, I was actually looking forward to the operation.

I remember being rolled on the stretcher into the operating room. The anesthesiologist started marking up my scalp. I got nervous as I thought of infamous surgical mishaps, like a patient going in to have the right foot amputated but having them cut off the left by mistake. This was not about to happen to me. I cried out in panic, "What are you doing in my head?" He gently replied, "I'm marking the places that will help us to connect you to the computer. This will help us determine that we have tested all the parts so that when we wake you all your body parts will function properly." I replied, "Mark on!" I do not remember much more after that as the anesthesia kicked in.

When I regained consciousness, I heard myself saying, "Thank you Jesus," over and over. I was thankful, I was awake. Thank you Jesus. I recall someone saying, "We need you to be quiet Krystal." I don't know if I stopped but if I did, I know it was still in my heart, "Thank you Jesus." They moved me into a dark room where I drifted in and out of sleep. I vaguely remember the surgeon coming in to check on me. He wanted me to raise my foot up off the bed. It was a simple request but how difficult it was! My foot felt heavy. "Did it move? Why is this so hard? I know. I'm still too drugged to fulfill the doctor's request. I'll do it later, Doc."

When I woke again, there was a nurse at my side and the room was still very dark. I imagine I was very low to the floor because I could see night lights which seemed to be at the base of the other beds. In the center of the room was a nurses' station. I watched the nurses move about doing I suppose what nurses do. From my bed, I could see a man walking towards the nurses' station. I could see clearly that he was carrying the most beautiful bouquet of flowers. They were not just beautiful but unusually gorgeous. Someone was going to be really happy to receive such a lovely array of flowers. Then I heard the man ask for Mrs. Gill. Were those flowers for me? Was I the only Gill in the area? If the flowers were so beautiful in the dark, I could not wait to see them in the light. I did not have to wait long. One of the nurses came and turned on the light. To my delight, they were from my brother and his wife in Texas. That night I had visitors coming just to see the flowers. They were beautiful. I guess the chant now is, "Pink, pink, *you're not sooo bad?*"

I stayed in that part of the hospital until I was told that I was going to be part of an acute rehab program for people with spinal cord injuries (SCI). Although I would be a long way from home, I felt remaining in the same hospital was a good idea because I had already come so far with the medical team. Why change locations when things were working well? I began my day with breakfast and a sponge bath. This was followed by occupational therapy (OC), physical therapy (PT), and recreational therapy. These were the most intense four hours! Thank goodness for a rest period and lunch. I am happy to report that my therapy began on a Thursday and by Friday I was not defeated. I was actually more encouraged to know that eventually I was going to walk. Amy, my physical therapist, helped me take my first steps and I could see she was as determined as I was. That night, I made a mental note to request a journal to record my progress.

By Saturday, I was glad there was a break from OC and PC. Therapy was not easy. It was both physically and emotionally draining. Couple that with stubborn body parts that wouldn't perform as I wanted them to… it was tough. I was tired. Like many people who work during the week, I wanted to sleep in on Saturday morning. But I had promised Allison, my social worker, that I would come to her recreation segment. It seemed like forever getting dressed that morning. I needed so much assistance and I still had to wait to be helped into the wheelchair and rolled to the recreation lounge. Nevertheless, Allison sent word that she and the other patients would wait for me.

The game we played was Allison's version of "The Price Is Right." We played the first game and I won. How fitting. The challenges to getting to the recreation room were worth it! And an unexpected bonus: there were prizes! As Allison showed me the prize collection from which I could choose, I could not believe what I saw: a pink journal! That was the moment I decided the name of my journey, **Rethinking Pink**.

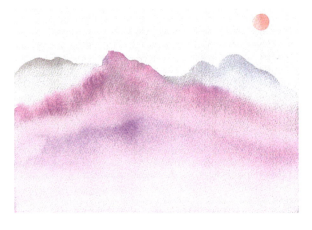

Chapter 2:

RETHINKING REST

And he said unto me, My grace is sufficient for thee: for my strength is made perfect in weakness. Most gladly therefore will I rather glory in my infirmities, that the power of Christ may rest upon me.

(2 Corinthians 12:9)

Go with the flow. Take time to smell the roses. You get the idea. Relax. I have always been told that you never know what is going to happen from one moment to the next. I had asked my husband, Joseph, if I could work late to catch up on paperwork at school. I had cooked dinner the day before and I thought I could work at least until seven that evening. In his usual agreeable way, he said sure. But when the day was over, I changed my mind. I wanted to be home with the two most important people in my world. My husband and my son had just returned the night before from a cruise they had taken with my in-laws. I was telling myself to go home and relax so I could listen to them share the details of their trip. I remember pulling a chair toward me so I could sit down and turn off the computer but that is not what happened. Somehow the chair escaped my grasp. Before I realized it, I fell, hitting the windowsill behind me and the computer desk in front of me. I lay on the floor not sure if I was alright but too scared not to act as if I were.

Because my classroom housed the afterschool program, it was full of children and adults. I was quickly attended to by the school nurse. In fact, there were two of them due to the transition period. They wanted to help me up but I felt like I just needed to lie still. The principal called my home and told me my husband was on the way. When he arrived about 20 minutes later, he helped me up. I was glad that the nurse let me take my time and wait for Joseph. I could tell that something was really wrong, but I did not know how to verbalize my concern. I wanted to get to the other school to set up my morning classes for the rest of the week. I wanted to think that this was not really happening and that I did not need to go to an emergency room. I wanted to go home and have dinner with my guys. To my chagrin, not only was I at a special care unit, but then I had to be attended to at an actual hospital emergency room. My night as I had planned it was over.

The attending doctor at the emergency center was being cautious that I had not fractured my neck. I wished that they would hear me and take care of the awful pain in my head. With medication and three days off for rest, I was discharged from the hospital and able to go home. Resting is a strange concept for me. I am usually on the go from the time I get up until I almost fall into bed. I rested those three days. I got up in the morning, came downstairs and did nothing. I could tell that I was not myself. I had to take extended time. I remember calling the emergency room to tell them that I had not received a doctor's follow-up call. I spoke to a lady who cared enough to secure a visit before the end of the next week. The doctor I saw did not think I was in the right place. He sent me to a pain management specialist. I learned that I had a concussion, occipital neuralgia and needed therapy to help eliminate the stiffness and pain I had in turning my neck from side to side.

As the days and weeks went by, I became anxious. When could I go back to work? Was all that I was experiencing due to a fall? How many more doctor visits would it take? How much more therapy? Why now? But still the voice in my ear would whisper, "Everything is all right, Krystal. Just rest." In the meantime, all I could do was rest. And there was plenty of pain killers and muscle relaxers to help me along the way. I was so groggy that there were times I had to be awakened to go to therapy. This was, to say the least, out of the ordinary for me. I was used to jet setting all around town and that was every day, including weekends.

My weekday routine had changed. Normally the day would begin with me waking at the usual hour as though I were getting ready for work. But since I could not go to work, I would try to make my son's lunch and send him off. I used to have the privilege of taking him to school on my way to work. It was only a few minutes but in that time my teenager could reveal more than he would if we were home all day. I would then try my therapy exercises while waiting for my husband to come home from his work on the night shift. Together we would have breakfast and somewhere between eating and listening to the televangelists I would fall asleep.

Life is strange when your head is hurting. Nevertheless, I took comfort in listening to the message of the televangelists. Every day it was as though they were telling me to rest in the love of God. How the message would resonate in my spirit! Just when I might feel a little too anxious, another message would come to calm me. Can you imagine how it feels to have such peace and unconditional love flowing all around you at a time when you are feeling so helpless and vulnerable? At times my fall seemed surreal, as though I was in a situation but not really there. There were times when I thought I should be able to get up in the morning and go to work and do the things I did from day to day that I once took for granted. When this would happen, I would get very still and talk to God. I would let go and share my concerns, my fears, and try to reach the root of my anxiety. And that's when I heard the Spirit ask, "Krystal, do you really love me?"

One thing I have learned in my Christian walk is that if the Spirit asks me a question, my immediate response is not necessarily the answer I believe but rather an answer that I would hope to respond. It was about this time that I heard an old hymn that has truly become strength in my weakness. I particularly like the version performed by Steve Green, a contemporary gospel artist.

Jesus, I Am Resting, Resting[1]
By Steven Chapman

Jesus, I am resting, resting
In the joy of what Thou art
I am finding out the greatness
Of Thy loving heart
Thou has bid me gaze upon Thee
And Thy beauty fills my soul
For by Thy transforming power
Thou has made me whole

O, how great Thy loving kindness
Vaster, broader than the sea!

---

[1] Green, Steven. Jesus, I Am Resting, Resting. Apple Music, 2010, Accessed July 28, 2022.

O, how marvelous Thy goodness
Lavished all on me!
Yes, I rest in Thee Beloved
Know what wealth of grace is Thine
Know Thy certainty of promise
And have made it mine

REFRAIN
Jesus, I am resting, resting
In the joy of what Thou art
I am finding out the greatness
Of The loving heart

Ever lift Thy face upon me
As I work and wait for Thee
Resting 'neath Thy smile, Lord Jesus
Earth's dark shadows flee
Brightness of my Father's glory
Sunshine of my Father's face
Keep me ever trusting, resting
Fill me with Thy grace

REFRAIN

I am finding out the greatness of Thy loving heart

I began playing this song over and over throughout the day. I played it when I got up in the morning and it was the last thing I heard before I fell asleep at night. I started thinking about what it means to rest. A natural rest is relaxing from work. In conversations with my mother, she would tell me how my father was truly in a state of rest. He was doing absolutely nothing but eating and sleeping. Well at the time, my father had very serious health issues that were making it difficult for him to do much.

I have learned and witnessed that in many instances, when a woman says she is doing nothing, she is cleaning, cooking, shopping or attending to a matter that is necessary in the daily course of household normalcy. On the other hand, when a man says he is doing nothing, nothing is what he is doing. So in my attempt as a woman to do nothing, I fell into a state of overwhelming fatigue. It was amazing to find out that I could not fix a complete meal for my family or do the wash or some of the other household chores that were once done without a second thought. And thinking, that is another area where in order to relax I was expected to turn off the flooding brain flow that was ever telling me of the chores and tasks that needed to be done and were far from being accomplished.

Up until I heard the song, I could not naturally rest. As I began to let the words minister to me, bit by bit I could hear what the televangelists were saying. There is a rest that comes when we understand how much God loves us. I can get caught up in thinking that what I do is how I pay my way into my family. In some respect, I believed that my housework was what enabled me to continue contributing proportionately into my family. But I was not thinking how God wanted me to think. God wanted me to cast all my cares on him. He wanted me to take no thought of tomorrow for tomorrow would take care of itself. To understand that I was in a period of time where doing nothing was doing the will of God in order to heal myself in body and in spirit was what some would call a *wow* moment. I was beginning to believe that I was loved in spite of my limitations and inabilities. This led me to the profound awareness of spiritual rest. In His way, God was letting me know that I needed His peace, a place of calm above my circumstance in which I placed my head in His hands. As I allowed myself to rest in the Lord, I could hear the Spirit telling me that all is well. My love for God and my willingness to obey Him was all that mattered. I did not have to focus on my situation for I was learning it was merely an attempt to distract me from where I was being led spiritually. What an awesome sensation to know that in relaxing, I was truly in the hands of God.

Neither my husband nor my son insisted that I do anything. In fact, their ability to step up to the plate and do the things I would normally do revealed their compassion toward me. Joseph would complete his night job shift to have to take me directly to an appointment or therapy. We struggled with whether or not appointments should be made in the morning or after he had had a chance to rest. Sometimes we did not have a choice. He was now the sole driver in our family which meant we also needed him to drive my son around to baseball, boy scouts and whatever else came up. All of which I used to do while he was sleeping. I could see my condition taking a toll on him, but he was driven by a conviction that my situation was going to get better. We were going to go to every therapy session to make it happen!

I watched my son Julius mature in many ways. He had always been able to get up and get ready for school on his own. As teens grow however, what they once did can sometimes fade away. I am grateful to say that for the rest of that school year, Julius was either on the bus or made it his business to walk to school, on time, each day. I could have felt left out for the times I wanted to go to the school concerts to hear him play his trumpet or watch him play baseball or take part in other social events, but the key was to rest as my husband took over. How amazing it was to have the love of two wonderful men rooting for me.

Complications arose with my back that required surgery in the Fall of 2015. The operation was scheduled for October 7th at Strong Hospital in Rochester. It was supposed to be a five day stay at the most. By this time, I was okay with the path that I was on. I could feel that God was with me, carrying me. I truly felt as though He had lavished His goodness upon me. The natural rest I had had for almost a year had quieted my inner spirit and I was beginning to feel whole. While in prayer with my prayer partner, I heard the Spirit say, "When you come out of the operation, you will have your ministry." What an inspiration that was as I went through with the operation. I could not wait to see what kind of mission a person could have after an operation.

Well, as I said before, after the operation, my lower body did not move. I thought that I was drugged and in a sense that meant that my body was still resting. I was told I had a spinal cord injury, and I was detained at the hospital for a month. Some might think that this was horrible. I saw it as God telling me to continue resting in Him. In a hospital bed unable to do for myself, completely dependent upon the workers for assistance, I was rested enough to know that just like the song said, I was resting underneath the smile of the Lord Jesus in a hospital room where many might have considered paralysis a dark shadow. In my room however, the shadows were all gone. The rest that I had found was a trust in Him so that I could encourage others. The brightness of my Father's glory and the sunshine of my Father's face had made it so that I could trust Him and rest in knowing that I was coming through the hospital ordeal.

When I returned home in early November, I still had to rest naturally. I wanted to show off that I could easily move around. But there I was, in a temporary hospital bed, unable to walk far from it. I told myself to rest because every day was a day of gaining strength. The initial home visits from my therapists gave Joseph his own much needed rest for which I was glad. I needed him to help me get dressed in the morning and to prepare my breakfast, but by the new year, we started thinking about how to ask others for help in transporting me to doctors' appointments and therapy sessions. Thank goodness for biological and spiritual sisters.

Although my desire to take Julius on a long college tour the summer of 2016 was squashed, he instead learned to drive. This was so important to us because we had agreed that he could attend the community college rather than completing his senior year at the high school. To accomplish this, Julius had to be able to transport himself. He passed his driver's test and was able to take himself to every one of his classes. And God, in His merciful way, gave us mild winter weather for Syracuse. You may wonder whether I was anxious about him being a novice driver. As a parent of course I would have been if I had let my mind go that way. I chose instead to rest in the daily prayers I prayed and told God "thank you" every time I saw my son return home safely.

Reports on the news and in the magazines, I read are constantly saying how little rest Americans get each day. The world is constantly telling us how we need to know what is happening all the time. Twenty-four-hour television and news, social media and the Internet all aid in keeping us knowledgeable of the sense and nonsense around us. There are reports in the news about cell phone addiction. People can hardly go on vacation without detaching themselves from the possibility of missing a call. Many people sleep with their cell phone within reach. News reports emphasize the importance and health benefits of uninterrupted sleep. Nevertheless, many of us do not heed such warnings. But Jesus said, *"Come unto me all ye that labour and are heavy laden, and I will give you rest." (Matthew 11:28)*

Remember to rest. No matter what condition you are in you will be better off if you rest. Rest provides the strength we need to conquer the challenges of the day. Furthermore, and perhaps more importantly, rest is the time when the Spirit can speak to our souls and provide the comfort and the answers we need to continue on our journey. No one is greater than God. He rested on the seventh day. Christ Jesus did too. Rest your cell phone too. Imagine the dinner table as a place for family conversation, reaching out to one another, for problem solving and showing that we care for one another. In this way you will bring a peace to your home that is often overlooked. Tell yourself and your family how much more meaningful they are than the cellphone and watch the benefits you will receive. And if you can, then understand Jesus wants us to experience his peace on a higher, deeper level. If you cannot sincerely say, "Jesus, I am resting, resting in the joy of who you are; I am finding out the greatness of your loving heart," keep repeating it until you can.

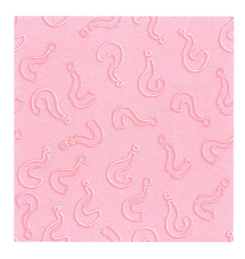

Chapter 3:

RETHINKING 'WHY ME?'

"For I know the thoughts that I think toward you, saith the Lord, thoughts of peace, and not of evil, to give you an expected end."
(Jeremiah 29:11)

If you were to look in the newspaper or watch the news, there just doesn't seem to be an answer to explain why catastrophe happens. Sometimes, as the reporter or announcer tells the story, there is even a gasp as the brain tries to process horrific information and gory details. Sometimes the information is so unbearable that the immediate reaction is to stop reading or change the channel. Occasionally, a period of thought-paralysis sets in as the mind cries out this is just too much to process. Stories of missing children, theft, car crashes, murder, misconduct, etc. are questioned and discussed among family members, friends and even co-workers. All too often the mind is trying to understand, empathize and imagine the devastation that occurred.

Unlike these events, my experience would not qualify for a feature in the newspaper or the plot of a made-for-TV docudrama. Nevertheless, when I think back, I realize it could have been viewed as a horrific situation. I was caught in what seemed to be a never-ending cycle of doctors, therapists and medication, all of which had a common goal, to eliminate the consequences of a fall that had suddenly changed my life. Independence as I once knew it was now redefined. Driving independently no longer existed. Freedom to move and do as I pleased was now subject to the availability, desire and convenience of others, assuming I was willing to ask.

When a person falls, usually they just get back up. This time wasn't like any of my previous falls. I couldn't just shake it off. From this fall, I suffered severe pain in my neck, head and eyes. Frequent muscle spasms were a noted side effect from the muscle relaxers. But I was not only suffering from the fall. After surgery, my affliction included recovering from the spinal cord injury (SCI). I had to learn to walk again, a process that included more complications than I could have imagined. There was the back brace I had to wear, and a hover mat apparatus that the aids had to use to transfer me from the bed to the chair and the walker. I can't tell you how much therapy I received in the acute ward. Classified as occupational, physical and social therapy, I was daily engaged during my extended hospital stay. The physical and emotional exhaustion left me only too happy to see the weekend come, even though there was therapeutic homework which the nurses made sure you completed. All this I endured while over an hour away from home. And if what I stated was not enough, I also gained an incredible amount of weight as a side effect of the medication, limited movement and inflammation: that all made personal hygiene quite challenging.

During the first year, I was constantly thinking I needed to rest. It seemed to keep my mind off the amount of medication I had to take to endure the pain. After the surgery, I thought I needed the rest to be able to fully participate in the therapy the spinal cord injury required. In the initial weeks after spinal surgery, to wake up and realize that the body is not functioning as it ought to, is frightening. Why is this happening to me? But that was not my first thought. The first night, I realized that two of my toes were moving. I remember saying, "Lord, you said that after the surgery my ministry would begin. So I thank you for having the activity of my toes. I look forward to what you are going to allow me to do tomorrow. Good night."

When the doctors made their rounds the next morning, I could move a few more of my toes and then the game began. The more I thanked God for the ability to move what I could with the strength He gave me from day to day, the more I seemed to accomplish. I now had an appreciation for rest. I was eager to go to bed each night to say, "thank you" and to see what the new day would bring. First my toes moved. From there, I was able to lift my foot up in the air higher and higher each day; not much, but noticeably.

Within a week my doctors recommended I move to the acute therapy ward. I had no idea what I was in for, but I was committed to doing the best I could to improve my condition. I was moved in on a Thursday evening and Friday afternoon there was a young therapist standing behind me pushing my legs forward between the parallel bars. I was standing on my feet and in motion again! What tears of joy flowed from my eyes that afternoon! I was so excited I thought I would stay up all night just praising and thanking God. The truth, I could barely keep my eyes open. A lot of energy is used up in therapy. By the time I was on my feet, I had to wait until late that evening before I could share with Joseph the joy of my progress.

Joseph! It was now past the time he had taken off to be with me during my surgery and recovery. He had arranged to stay at the hotel that gave him employee perks. Unfortunately, he had to vacate the premises when my stay was extended. There was a special boarding house dedicated for patients' families nearby where he dwelt a few days. As my convalescence stretched on, he had to return to Syracuse, back to work, back to our son. I did not think about how our life would be with me in Rochester and him in Syracuse. I did not even have a cell phone glued to my ear, as is the norm for so many these days. I had my room phone, and I had to wait for him to wake up after his night shift and call me. One thing I was always thinking about was the cost of extras. If we had lived in Rochester, our phone calls would have been free.

In truth, I knew that the distance between us was not easy for either of my guys. Joseph was becoming more and more exhausted. He would arrive home from work, take a nap and try to make it up in time for visiting hours to visit me. Sometimes upon arrival he would fall asleep on my bed. On those days he would leave in time to get home, take a shower and go to work. After 22 years of marriage, I knew this was no easy feat for him. He never was a night owl. We were trying to discuss how to change his night shift position before my initial fall. I say all this to say that it is no surprise when I learned from him about the conversations he would have with the Lord as he drove to and from the hospital. For Joseph the question "Why me?" came without an answer. Yet, I can remember standing in the back of the church we attend with the recently appointed pastor and assistant pastor. I was doing what I had been taught, informing them that I would have to go into the hospital. Joseph was standing there with me. The pastor said, "We will be praying for you." I responded, "I'll be just fine. Please pray for my husband's strength." They remarked as men do that I was the apple of his eye and that they understood his concern for me. But honestly, I meant it and reiterated, "Please pray for my husband's strength."

I was not just a wife out of commission but a mother also. Joseph had to concern himself with my needs, his needs and the needs of Julius, our son. Originally Markell, one of his older friends was going to stay in our house and keep him company. Five days became a month. Both guys were a good distraction for my husband. Julius told him of the football wins and losses from week to week and Markell challenged him to create wholesome meals that the young man would eat. Together they kept him thinking of ways to prevent our home from becoming a musty locker room. I had to laugh when Joseph showed me the extra hamper placed in the spare room Markell occupied. Thank goodness for my younger sister. She can clean up a mess faster than anyone I know, and she stopped by before I returned home to make the space habitable again.

They say every woman needs a daughter. Honestly, I am grateful for the son that I have. He can cook, clean, launder and get himself to and from school and football practice without parental assistance. His greatest contribution was knowing I would want him to do what was expected of him and not use my condition as an excuse to act out. Nevertheless, Julius also asked the question "Why?" Once in the hospital while he was visiting, he said, "Mom, you're the nicest person I know. Why would anyone want to hurt you?" After I had been home a while, he let me know that he was not pleased that I was still not myself. I could see the tears swelling in his eyes as I tried to get him to talk about the situation our family faced. Like his dad, the time was not yet for him to understand why.

One day in an attempt to get Joseph to say something about how he was handling our road bump, he instead played the songs below on his tablet.

When It Was Over[2]
by Sara Grove

When it was over and they could talk about it
She said there's just one thing I have got to know
What in that moment when you were running so hard and fast
Made you stop and turn for home
He said I always knew you loved me even though I'd broken your heart
I always knew there'd be a place for me to make a brand new start
Oh love wash over a multitude of things
Love wash over a multitude of things
Love wash over a multitude of things
Make us whole
When it was over and they could talk about it
They were sitting on the couch
She said what on earth made you stay here
When you finally figured out what I was all about

He said I always knew you'd do the right thing
Even though it might take some time
She said, Yeah, I felt that and that's probably what saved my life
Oh love wash over a multitude of things
Love wash over a multitude of things
Love wash over a multitude of things
Make us whole
There is a love that never fails
There is a healing that always prevails

---

[2] Groves, Sara. *When It Was Over*. Capitol Christian Music Group, Music Services, Inc, 2005, Accessed July 28, 2022.

There is a hope that whispers a vow
A promise to stay while we're working it out
So come with your love and wash over us

    I was sitting on the chair trying to keep from becoming a wet mess because I was beginning to understand the pain that Joseph had had to embrace. While in my heart I knew he was not leaving me, the separation we had was more real than I had imagined. We had existed without the other for a month and it had been no small feat. Although I was often too tired to think about being without him, I also knew that his world was completely upside down. The depth of pain was more than he had wanted to experience. Yet for me, I was able to mask the separation by cheering on others. I often would encourage other patients in therapy that would say they wanted to go home. I told them they had to make the most of their stays, and the professional assistance at their disposal because when they got back home, they wouldn't have so much help. I was clandestinely encouraging myself. These thoughts flowed through my mind as the song above played. And then Joseph played the song below.

Loving A Person[3]
By Sara Groves

Loving a person just the way they are, it's no small thing
It takes some time to see things through
Sometimes things change, sometimes we're waiting
We need grace either way
Hold on to me

---

[3] Groves, Sara. Loving A Person Brown Eyed Blonde Publishing, 2005, Accessed July 28, 2022

I'll hold on to you
Let's find out the beauty of seeing things through
There's a lot of pain in reaching out and trying
It's a vulnerable place to be
Love and pride can't occupy the same spaces baby
Only one makes you free
Hold on to me
I'll hold on to you
Let's find out the beauty of seeing things through
If we go looking for offense
We're going to find it
If we go looking for real love
We're going to find it

    This guy is no doubt the most romantic man I know. He is sensitive, kind, tenderhearted and I am trying to figure out how did I end up with the wonderful blessing of him. I can only believe that the awesome loving God I know loves me so much. Remember I said that when the accident occurred I could feel the love of the Lord as He wrapped me in His arms to remind me of His great love for me? I felt the essence of this same sentiment as I listened to the song play. I felt safer than I had ever felt with my love before. Just imagine being told that I need you so much that I would never want to let you go, that you could not bear to have anything separate one from the other. It reminded me of the decree that says:

> *Who shall separate us from the love of Christ? Shall tribulation, or distress, or persecution, or famine, or nakedness, or peril, or sword?... Nay, in all these things we are more than conquerors through him that loved us. For I am persuaded, that neither*

> *death, nor life, nor angels, nor principalities, nor powers, nor things present, nor things to come, nor height, nor depth, nor any other creature, shall be able to separate us from the love of God, which is in Christ Jesus our Lord. (Romans 8: 35, 37-39)*

And as the song ended and the next song began, I realized that I was once again in the presence of a man with mixed emotions. Twenty-five years earlier when he realized he loved me, he gave me a mixed tape he entitled "Blue Valentines," an array of songs expressing how frazzled I had caused him to become. This was a similar experience, where his music choices still expressed some tension. And yet he was also being compelled to think about something he had never considered before, the sovereignty of God.

What I Thought I Wanted[4]
By Sara Groves

Tuxedo in the closet, gold band in a box
Two days from the altar she went and
called the whole thing off
What he thought he wanted,
what he got instead
Leaves him broken and grateful
I passed understanding a long,
long time ago
And the simple home of systems
and answers we all know
What I thought I wanted,
what I got instead

---

[4] Groves, Sara. What I thought I Wanted 2004, Accessed July 28, 2022.

Leaves me broken and
Somehow peaceful
I keep wanting you to be fair
But that's not what you said
I want certain answers to these prayers
But that's not what you said
When I get to heaven
I'm gonna go find Job
I want to ask a few hard questions,
I want to know what he knows
About what it is he wanted and
what he got instead
How to be broken and faithful
What I thought I wanted (4x)
Staring in the water
like Esops foolish dog
I can't help but reflect on
what it was I almost lost
What it was I wanted, what I got instead
Leaves me broken and grateful
I'm broken and grateful
I want to be broken and grateful
I want to be broken, peaceful, faithful, grateful, grateful (2x)

Quietly and pensively Joseph and I shared the moment. Tears streamed down his face. Before I could ask, he gave me the lyrics he had already printed out. I later added them to the pink journal that held all the special moments of my experience and thanked Sarah Groves for writing what was so difficult to express.

Do we ever know the answer to why we go through pain, suffering, or separation? Only when we look to Christ Jesus can we begin to understand to suffer is to be put in position to live with Him. Our suffering helps to make us strong in our belief that we are more than conquerors through Christ who loves us. In our trials we can assess how much we fully rely on God to carry us through. The truth is we are only as alone as we want to be. So, when we are alone and feeling despair, then we must believe that He is there to carry us through. We go through by believing that the One who loves us more than anyone else, cares more than anyone else, pains more than anyone else, is never going to leave us alone.

I am not saying that this is as easy to believe or comprehend as I have written these words on the page. Nevertheless, I have learned that I can do all things through Christ who strengthens me. When I think why me, I believe it is because I have come to realize just how much God loves me. He is confident that I will love Him despite the challenges that the situation brings. But also, because, I had been prepared that something was going to happen. A relationship with God not only means that He is going to be by our side but that He has every detail sorted out. For me that meant there were no coincidences not even the name of the hospital or the large presence of international workers on the floor. What do I mean? Well, for starters, the name of the hospital is "Strong." The name is so significant to me because it is the name of my college residence hall. It was an all-women's residence in which I felt surrounded by powerful women who made me feel as though I could conquer any task or situation. Some of the matters

I conquered solely but others I conquered with the help of the sisterhood found within the walls of Strong. Hence it was a connection to something familiar, that gave me the feeling that things would work out.

I also appreciated the fact that so many of the workers were from countries outside the U.S.A. The study of culture, its people and places has always been a delight for me. I love learning languages and customs and just discovering how things are similar and different from one place to another. As I often say, God made a big, beautiful world and I want to see it all. Perhaps I won't physically experience it all, but the conversations I had at Strong Hospital allowed me to speak Spanish, some French and learn to say my numbers in Yemeni and Arabic. The language learning helped me to repeat the exercises I had to do without becoming monotonous and even utilize my teaching skills as my therapists would count along after me. As I look at the experience, I was actually having fun! What a thought! I was enjoying myself in the midst of a health crisis. Could I say I found peace in the midst of a storm?

There were also day-to-day hints that God was right beside me. In particular, I loved to hear the woman come in to freshen up my room. She was always singing the loveliest song in French. I could not catch all the words because my French has weakened since my college days. I tried to get her to write the words down for me, but this was met with a humble refusal. While I did not understand her reluctance, I enjoyed the sweetness in her voice as she would sing it almost every time I saw her. How happy my day seemed to be when I heard her. She finally told me it was a song expressing God's role in the creation of the world. I knew there was a reason for the melody to be so beautiful.

"Why me? More times than I care to enumerate, I find myself asking why not me. I can only think on the blessings I have received since the beginning of my pink experience. More importantly to me is how many times have I through this experience been a blessing to others. I loved to hear the workers as they told me the matters most dear to their heart and then to see them smile as we prayed together, or I gave words of encouragement. I derived great pleasure from seeing other patients gain strength as I cheered them on in the therapy room. I learned to wheel myself around the ward floor to visit other patients in their room. And although my husband and son were without me for a moment, they did not fall apart. God gave them grace and mercy as they tried to maintain order while I was away. He gave them strength to carry on and perks along the way. But that is their testimony to share.

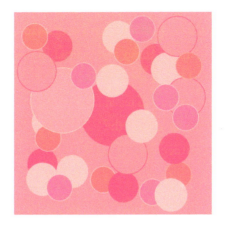

Chapter 9:

RETHINKING COMMUNITY

If it be possible, as much as lieth in you, live peaceably with all men.

(Romans 12:18)

Did you ever have a song that you just couldn't get out of your head? That is what happened to me. I remember when the song *I Need You To Survive* by Hezekiah Walker came out in 2002. Everybody was singing it, swaying to the beat, greeting each other with a smile and putting all the emphasis on the refrain "I need you to survive." Who knew that the words of Hezekiah Walker would play out so vividly in my life? There I was in the hospital more helpless than I could ever remember being. After the operation, I was able to move from the waste up. That meant I was able to move my arms, feed myself, talk on the phone and read. I needed assistance to do anything that required some form of mobility. I had to learn to roll over from one side of the bed to be assisted in daily toiletry and maintaining hygiene. I dressed my upper torso and waited for assistance to complete dressing. I was air lifted into a chair in order not to become too weakened from lying in bed. Later I had to learn to slide to the edge of the bed to be helped into the chair, to sit up for the day. Eventually I improved enough to be escorted to the bathroom, although I still needed full assistance to take care of business.

Now unless you too have been taught to guard your body for your spouse and to be careful how you present yourself in the presence of others, you cannot imagine the devastation I felt knowing that there were men everywhere around me. Yet, in the state I was in, there was no point acting as though I did not need the assistants and nurses to help me along the way. Literally, I needed every nurse and assistant to survive. I cannot begin to tell you the horror I felt the first time I rang for assistance and a male nurse came in to help me. Honestly, I wanted to cry. Surely the man at my side was a mistake. I mean, when they read my chart, did they not see that I am a woman, not a man? In an instant I had to decide whether I appreciated the help that I had been sent. So quickly I realized: the human body is merely an object to those who work in health care. While the workers learn to be sensitive to the needs of their patients, my naked body was merely of clinical interest. Nurses are taught to address the need and move on to the next. And so, in that moment, I told the male nurse what I needed, and my need was instantly met.

My respect for the community of male attendants gave me the ability to have my needs met more quickly than if I had opted for only females. I did not realize at the time that this gave me a reputation as being an easy patient, one that was not hostile and allowed the workers to do their job freely. I was not a needy patient. My greatest concern was trying to avoid wetting myself. I realized from a previous hospital stay that the closer you are to the nurses' station, the more attentive the caretakers were for your welfare. When I arrived on the acute therapy ward, I was first. But my reputation allowed the nurses to come see me as a means of "taking a break." Hence, I got more company than I needed. But when I did need attention, it seemed as though every worker on the floor rushed to my aid. Although I would never have said it out loud, I truly felt like a royal child.

I remember two incidences in particular. In the first situation, I needed to use the bathroom. I was not yet allowed to go on my own for fear that I would fall. But when you have to go, you have to go. I was feeling stronger and felt as though I could make it the short distance from the bed to the bathroom. I actually made it safely! Yet within moments, I could tell that something was not quite right. I was light-headed, so I had to call for assistance. I wasn't going to succeed in my sneaky attempt to be independent. The first person to arrive on the scene was one of the tallest men on staff. He was a friendly, familiar face. I remember liking him immediately. He had changed my sheets the day after I arrived. He had found a blue printed pillowcase that reminded him of something I said that I liked. I thought it was kind of him to want me to feel comfortable even down to the pillow I would rest my head on. We would have lots of endearing conversations during my stay. Anyway, in that moment, he was the best face I could have seen because I believed no one else would have had the strength to support my body, as enormous as I felt at the time. There he stood telling me not to worry; he had me and he would not let me fall. And he did this all while beckoning help from others to come and find out what was the matter with Mrs. Gill. Several men and women came. I was cleaned and taken back to bed. Sometimes even when you are doing well, a slight relapse can occur. When it happens, you just have to rest.

Another time, I was having occupational therapy in my room. I was so excited because I was finally going to get a full body shower. I was walked from my room to the shower around the corner. As I began to get undressed, I felt a wave of heat that was making me feel weak. I remember the therapist telling me to wait here on the seat in the shower and she was going for help. I do not remember anything else until I heard the head nurse call my name. I was on the floor in the hallway looking up to a lot of faces. With a smile I remember saying, "I guess something happened." I had passed out for the first time in my life. How fortunate, I thought at the time, to have so many people willing and ready to assist me in a time of need. I learned later that I was having episodes of syncope.

These were incidents which made me ponder just who were these people with whom I was sharing a month of my life. I concluded that they were a genuine community. Of course, a hospital building might be located in a neighborhood. It may even have the word "community" included in its name, but outside of those who work there, how many of us think of the hospital as a community?

I checked with the online dictionary. It defined **COMMUNITY** as follows:

> *1. a group of people living in the same place or having a particular characteristic in common. 2. a feeling of fellowship with others, as a result of sharing common attitudes, interests, and goals.*

Upon entering the acute ward at the hospital, I had entered into a new community. I was given a team of therapists. I remember the first day meeting one of them who asked, "Whose team are you on? I want you to be on my team." Clearly, I had no idea what it meant to be on their team, but I can tell you this: Each person on my team had a name that began with the letter "A." My team consisted of the occupational therapist, Amanda; the physical therapist, Amy; and the social/emotional therapist, Allison. These phenomenal women worked with me daily to help me surpass the necessary goals to prepare to return home.

Many people spell my name with a "C". When I was very young, my mother told me my name was spelled with a "K" and not a "C" because she did not want me to think of myself as an average person. I was to always seek to be better than average at anything I did. Hence, I expected, especially in academics, to attain the highest mark. Now some may think that this was a dangerous setup for experiencing inevitable human failure. Actually, it helps me to think that I can accomplish anything and that a healthier approach to failure is that it only exists upon surrender. A's are the goal with proper adjustments along the way. With my A-team (Amanda, Ashley and Allison), I just knew I was in a community of excellence. We laughed, we sang, we pumped ourselves up as we pushed passed the pain and challenges of therapy. They did not want to let me down and I did not want to let them down. We believed in each other as we worked to reach our common goal. I cannot think back on my pink experience without applauding their dedication and commitment to my recovery.

The other patients were an integral part of the community. There were my roommates, who I knew were facing challenges comparable to or worse than mine. We were able to cheer for each other in therapy and support one another through the night. I will never forget the day that I finally figured out how to roll around in my wheelchair. I would be able to visit my neighbors and offer up conversation or a prayer, or just an ear to listen which was what I found I did best. It is amazing how much one needs to be reminded that things will not always be as they are, and to be reassured to take the time to work through the tasks outlined by the therapists. How encouraging it is to recognize the progress we made each day. It is true that some gave up and just wanted to go home. I felt sad for them because the hospital community is really there to help you. It has the techniques, the apparatuses and the 24-hour manpower to get you to the best place, before you have to be on your own.

One of my favorite moments of the day was when the meals were brought to my room. I liked the entire process of ordering food. You started by looking over the menu. Then you could either give the order to the young lady who came to record your choice for the day or call in your order later. It was then usually brought to you by a young person (a child to me by age comparison). I really believed the food department was insistent on hiring only persons who were of nice appearance and personality. They were always pleasant and smiling. Although they were in a hurry to make their deliveries, they were patient enough to make sure that the meal was correct and to bring ice or other amenities requested. It did not seem to matter whether it was breakfast, lunch or dinner, I looked forward to the pleasantries that would come from these young people. They would converse with me and tell me their plans for their future. I appreciated how this community chose to make the eating experience a welcomed one. Frankly, some institutional food can hinder physical recovery. I know I looked forward to my meals because I felt as though I was working so hard and worked up an appetite. It really was a moment to take a break. I will admit I let my love for apple pie get the best of me. A word of caution: think twice before telling yourself apple pie—or your particular food delight—is necessary every night. It can take longer than anticipated to break the habit or lose the additional weight.

You could always tell who was good at the job and who was new in the field. Every shift your vitals were taken. At first this is not a terrible thing but then your body starts to say it has endured enough pokes and made enough blood offerings. I remember one night when one of the nurses told me he was a vampire and that he could get anything to drain. I fooled him.

A phlebotomist specialist had to come. I did not mean to tarnish his reputation, but then did I really want to cooperate with a vampire? Another nurse tried in so many places that I had to laugh. I hope she did not get in trouble for all the black and blues that were left in the wake of her determination.

There were daily workers—such as the receptionists, nurses and assistants—who were vital to the success of my recovery. I enjoyed each interaction I had with them. I wish I could list each of the daily workers and tell you why they were so special to me. I am afraid someone would surely be forgotten and that would make me sad. I thank them for coming to talk to me and thereby establishing my sense of self-worth. I appreciated how they valued my perspective and counsel. Some would pray with me or let me pray for them. Some would let me tell them of my life experiences and share theirs. Some would tell of the most devastating matters that were happening to them at the time. I was always in awe that they would allow me to pour into their lives.

Of course, the doctors have had special significance for me. I have to admit that I don't want to be in the hands of any physician other than Jehovah Rapha *(God my Healer)*. Nevertheless, the doctors I met during this experience are like no other doctors I've known. I always felt that they were listening to me and that they heard everything I was saying. I did not feel rushed in their presence; I didn't even mind being observed by the student interns. This was major, as I remember being in the hospital once before, after the birth of my son, and I did not want to see any interns.

During my stay in Strong Hospital, I realized the necessity of allowing all the workers to do their part in assisting in my convalescence. In so doing, I reached my goal of returning home with confidence I would be alright. As an educator, I can only imagine the gains that could be reached in our schools, neighborhoods, governments, etc., if we really operated in harmony. What an awesome concept to discover—to come to the realization that I need you and you need me and that this applies to whatever community of which we are connected. How amazing it would be if each one felt important enough to help another person to survive. Would this not be the meaning of having God in our life and understanding His will: to meet the needs of one another?

    I do not want to ever believe that I am in this world alone. I want to remember that everything we experience can contribute to helping others in some manner. Either I am helping someone reach their goal or someone is helping me to reach mine. It warrants a concept of selflessness on the part of each individual that pushes another to be above average, where everyone can get an "A."

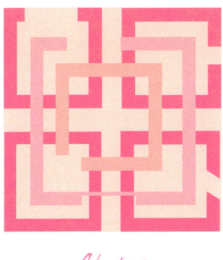

Chapter 5:

RETHINKING DISABILITY

Turn thee unto me and have mercy upon me; for I am desolate and afflicted.

(Psalm 25:17)

When I was an elementary student, my father had a friend who always asked, "Who's better looking, me or your dad?" I would laugh and reply every time, "My dad." I loved Mr. Thomas. He had an excellent sense of humor, and he never left the house without taking notice of me. He was an accountant who made me promise to take calculus before I stopped taking math courses. It was because of that promise that I took it twice: in Spain as a high school senior studying abroad, and then again, my freshman year of college. I received credit the first time because my classmates pleaded with the instructor to pass me. I passed well the second time around.

Mr. Thomas would have been pleased to know that I did not avoid the challenge of studying calculus. He had passed away by the time I went to Spain but that only gave me more determination. However, in the middle of my studies that year abroad, I remember thinking that I was crazy to stay in the class. The teacher had very little command of the English language and I had little command of Spanish. My classmates made me feel that I could get through the course with their assistance as their language ability was more fluent than mine. I chose not to drop the class, but I could never understand the instructor nor benefit from his numerous attempts to tutor me. I was lost even listening to my classmates as they conversed about the subject matter in and out of class.

Was comradery with these mathematical geniuses worth the inevitable agony I would feel when I received an "F" on my transcript? I mean, who does this knowing a poor grade could hinder getting into college. I began to worry that I wouldn't get into my college of choice. Prior to arriving in Spain, I was convinced that I wanted to go to a large university. I had applied to six universities and only one college, Vassar. I was beginning to feel that my college advisor, who recommended I not even apply to Vassar with my grades, was right.

When the term was ending, I recall how the instructor stood before the class and began to announce our marks. In that moment I dreaded the humiliation that I alone failed the class. The instructor looked at me and said in his language, "Krystal, I'm sorry I cannot pass you." Then one of my friends fell on his knees before the instructor in a begging position and told him that he was creating a great injustice. That we are a family and there was no way any of my peers would accept him failing me. The rest of the class responded with a wave of imploring that neither the professor nor I had ever expected. The result was that my grade was changed to a D and hence, I "passed." It was the sweetest "D" I had ever had. Of course, in the back of my mind was that I had failed and upon entering my freshman year at Vassar, it was a course I knew I *had* to retake.

Taking calculus twice was one of my greatest life lessons. It taught me that failure is the act of giving up on a particular situation. I believe Mr. Thomas knew this was true. He was a man that faced difficult challenges every day. As the result of a car crash, Mr. Thomas was a double leg amputee. He learned to get around with his wheelchair and lots of taxis. I'm not sure why he did not use prosthetics, but I know he embraced life. I loved knowing that he appeared to give no excuse for not doing what he needed to do to get where he needed to go.

I suppose Mr. Thomas helped me to receive another person I so admire but have never met personally. I have found great strength in the life of Joni Eareckson Tada. I heard her on the radio in the mid 80s and fell in love with her voice and her love for God. She made living for Him sound so easy, something that I too have always felt. I had been listening to Joni on the radio for quite a while before I learned her back story. After graduating from high school, she and her sister had gone swimming. She tried a dive that landed her in the hospital. The injuries left her a paraplegic. I remember hearing her tell her story of how it was cool to see so many people visiting her through the summer. The reality of her injuries did not hit her until her friends were heading off to college and she was still in the hospital.

Before you are discharged from the hospital, there are papers and instructions you are expected to follow, and prescriptions you need to fill. I think it was the paper that said I should request disability parking that made me begin to face reality. The truth however was that I did not apply for the little parking pass you hang on the rearview mirror indicating disability. I left the hospital during the cold month of November, and December was even colder. Winter in Central New York is too cold to care about going outside unless you love winter activities. And, I had home care through January. Hence, there was no reason to leave the house.

When Spring rolled around, I had outpatient physical therapy. Having had driving restrictions, I did not need the disability card because the kindness of my caretakers automatically placed me at the front door wherever I went. Most of them were caretakers of someone else and had their own disability parking pass. I did not mind using the walker as I was building myself up and I did not see the walker as a permanent necessity. Furthermore, I used my tall, strong husband and son as my canes. How I loved them for being there. But I was in denial. I did not want impaired legs. I could walk holding on to the wall at first and little by little I could let go and walk a distance without wall support. After some time, I could feel "normal' by using a shopping cart as my walker.

The difficulty for me was that with every gain I seemed to make, there would be an unforeseen setback causing me to feel as though I was starting the walking process anew. The summer after my surgery, I found a friend who accompanied me walking. We would stroll along Lake Onondaga, on a well-known local path enjoyed by joggers and cyclists. It was a place where over the years I had spent much time running or walking with other friends. My winter confinement left me without another walking partner until the following autumn. I met a neighbor who was willing to accompany me. Together we walked up and down the hills in our neighborhood. With my new-found friend beside me, I felt as though I could move on my own. My balance was better, but the challenge was still before me. All too soon, it was winter again.

Winter brings snow, ice and falls. A complication of my injury was my constant concern about falling. I could fall at any time, and for a while I could not pick myself up. I slowly learned some pointers on how to stand up after a fall. This is especially important to give my husband and son the confidence to allow me to be in the house alone. Getting up from a fall is painful. Once on the floor, it is necessary to use your knees and toes to roll over and prop yourself up. When I fall, there is not only soreness, but for some reason the nerves in my knees and toes couldn't bear the pressure. It took more time than I care to recall before I could endure the pain of being on my knees and pushing on my toes to get up.

My disability denial was also prolonged by my personal income. I was blessed to receive worker's compensation along with enough salary to not feel the sting of monetary loss. When the salary portion ended, I was still feeling secure because there were no major bills to pay, a wonderful benefit of obeying the voice of the Lord telling us to get rid of our credit card debt years ago. But in another sense, we were living from paycheck to paycheck. Our son was going to college as a high school senior; so there was a need for more income. As lawyers do for their clients, mine suggested I apply for disability services.

I received two letters declaring me permanently disabled: one by the workers' compensation board and the other from the State of New York. I can still feel the tear falling on my face. As I searched Google for a description of my present situation, I learned that the term handicapped means "someone has a permanent injury, illness, or other problem that makes them unable to use their body or mind normally." That description was not as polite as "disabled." Personally, I tell people that I am "afflicted," a biblical term meaning I am enduring a hardship. It is harder for me to walk, but I walk. It is harder for me to read for long periods of time, but I read. It is harder for me to concentrate without getting a headache, but I push myself to understand. So often, one can give up or resort to the expression, "I can't…" I have learned that *"I can do all things through Christ which strengthens me."* (Philippians 4:13) It just may take me a little longer or require the assistance of an apparatus.

My affliction forced me to retire from my teaching position sooner than I anticipated. I have not abandoned my desire to teach. I am so excited about exploring other possibilities of how and what to teach that I get more excited with each of the possibilities that come my way. One consideration I have had happened by going to a birthday party for a friend. She invited her guests to a paint party. This was not my first time attending such an event. This time however, I could see myself in the role of instructing the clients to paint the scenes on the canvases. As I continued to paint, I realized the teacher was doing exactly what I used to do except in a different setting and a different subject.

As a teacher, you can often get supply catalogs sent to your home. As I flipped through the latest catalog, I asked myself how would I justify purchasing the items I wanted to buy. Within a few days, I met a man in the store that told me of the school he and his wife started in West Africa. The summer past, they had a session where volunteers came to teach the students different languages. He asked if I wanted to come. Because I was standing behind a shopping cart, he could not see that I was afflicted. I gave him my testimony and he gave me an open invitation to come when I was ready. I am getting ready.

I am working toward the goal of being able to travel. Presently, my affliction makes traveling impractical but not impossible. Sitting too long causes unbearable stiffness. Hotel accommodations need to be considered in terms of the accessibility of the bed, the commode, the shower, etc. The hardest part of not being able to travel is that my parents live about a four-hour car drive, without stops. I used to take the trip without a second thought. Now, on a good day the trip to my doctor, an hour and fifteen minutes away, must be done with at least one rest stop. The first time since my affliction that I was driven home was a beautiful day. I had to recuperate for a day going and coming. Now each time I go it seems I experience less discomfort, although one can make the mind forget the actual suffering for the joy of seeing loved ones. I am encouraged that I will not only be a passenger but with car technology and disability apparatuses, I will one day be able to drive myself wherever I need to go.

There are many circumstances to be considered for a disabled person. I attended a social event for women at a museum. I laughed inside as I realized there was nothing for me to lean against in the main atrium. When I arrived, there was already a mass of women in the center of the room. Standing also were venders located against the wall. The food was in the center with a couple of stands already occupied by guests that had arrived before me. I had a walker (although not the kind with a seat attachment) and that helped a great deal. A friend brought a person who was confined to a wheelchair for mobility.

Unfortunately, some of the events were unable to be reached by wheelchair. I give the attendants credit for finding alternative means by which to take us from one floor to the next bypassing stairways, but clearly the needs of disabled participants were overlooked in committee preparation. Two of my chief concerns are why ramps to get into a building are usually so long and why the bathroom stall for wheelchair accommodation is usually the farthest from the entrance. Perhaps it is not so bad from a wheelchair, but walking can make life shaky if you are using a walker.

One day I saw from my backyard a fawn trying to jump the fence. I was wondering where the mother was. As I looked, I finally saw her on the other side laying low. After several attempts, the fawn seemed to give up. The mother jumped over and gave the fawn a little milk. She would not allow it to drink long. It was as though the fawn had received a pep talk and then back to the other side the mother went. I marvel at how God used this image to tell me, "You can do it." I cannot say that I cry so much. Occasionally, I find myself whimpering just like the fawn. Just like the fawn and its mother, God sends something or someone to encourage me along the way.

I have my greatest moments of encouragement when I thank God for the things I can do. So often I remember when I was in the hospital and I would praise Him for the fact that my toes were moving. Then little by little I had the ability to move my foot, and then my legs, up and down off the bed. Not much but a little. After arriving home, I heard Joyce Myers tell the story of one of her co-workers whose daughter had caught pneumonia and was in a vegetative state. Her parents were so focused on what she could not do they forgot to thank God for what she was able to do. The father told how Joyce Myers told him to start thanking God for what she could do and eventually, he and his family had the testimony of how his daughter went back to finish her studies at the university. For me the story was merely confirmation of what I believed I needed to do: give God my "anyhow" praise.

An "anyhow" praise is a praise that comes from the depth of your soul. It allows you to acknowledge that God is indeed sovereign. He is not unaware of the affliction of His people. In fact, as I have learned, He cares more deeply for those who realize they ought to fully rely on Him for He will supply every need especially in times of hardship. As a natural father would want to relieve the suffering of his child, so would my heavenly Father want to take me out of my affliction. How quickly we forget that He wanted us to live with Him always in the Garden of Eden. Nevertheless, some of us have the privilege to serve as object lessons for others because of our disabilities. Practice being kind, patient, and compassionate. In an interview with Joni Eareckson Tada commemorating 50 years as a disabled person she stated:

> *"People with disabilities bring … a great audiovisual aid of how to deal with hardship. They show … how God's power can be*

> *released through weakness, and we all need examples of that. We need to see people who are smiling and persevering and enduring through their hardships."* [5]

It often takes great effort to endure hardship. People do not often know how to act comfortably in one's presence. Sometimes words can come out that are disheartening or lacking sensitivity. I wonder sometimes if Mr. Thomas always spoke to calm my natural childlike inquisition as I stared at his amputated legs. His jovial manner really said, "I know who I am and I'd like for you to get to know me." That's how I felt. I am still the same Krystal I was before my afflictions and I love the Lord no less, perhaps a bit more. May God be glorified in me. I salute Mr. Thomas for his endearing laughter and his push to make me promise to study calculus. And I thank Joni Eareckson Tada for using the beauty of the voice God gave her to reach my heart and mind long before I knew I was in preparation to be so used by God. Another dear friend of mind that lived to be 99 years old once gave me these words of advice, "Embrace where you are in life and move forward." And so, I will.

---

[5] Eareckson, Tada. After 50 Years in a Wheelchair, I Still Walk with Jesus Interview by Kelli B. Trujillo| July 28, 2017.

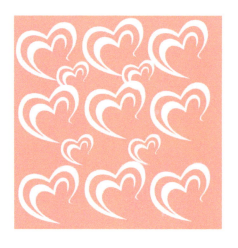

Chapter 6:

RETHINKING FEAR

Yea, though I walk through the valley of the shadow of death, I will fear no evil: for thou art with me; thy rod and thy staff they comfort me.

(Psalm 23: 4)

When it comes to fear, during the earliest years of my life, I was ruled by it. I feared bridges, roller coasters, dentists, failure, growing up, changes, being broke, hell, death, and dying. Merriam-Webster defines fear as "an unpleasant, often strong emotion caused by anticipation or awareness of danger." I walked with a spirit of darkness I could not explain nor shake away because I experienced fear in almost every situation. In essence, I even feared living. As a result, depression was my constant companion. Then one day, I committed my life to serving Christ Jesus. It was then I believed that I no longer felt such fears. Well, at least I didn't feel them as strongly. I still had my moments.

Let me give you an example. When I was young, I may have gone to the dentist a few times. Although biannual visits were recommended by most dentists, I had heard enough graphic stories of dental torment. I also knew that I had a few teeth that begged dental treatment that I did not allow anyone to know about. The desire to conceal my bad teeth, coupled with the fear caused by a reoccurring dream of my teeth coming out from the root, meant that I had to do everything possible to stay away from the dentist. The dentist was my childhood boogieman. Fear made me believe the dentist would take away my teeth, instead of helping me retain them. For years I walked around with both this fear and bad teeth.

As I got older, I found dentists with whom I was comfortable and gradually built enough confidence to take care of my major problems. Yet, for each established relationship I had with a dentist, I can also tell you a story about how relocation rekindled my dental fears. I'll only tell one of the many. Just before embarking on a two-year tenure as an English teacher in Japan, I had a dentist with whom I had learned to relax. I told the dentist to make certain that all the bridges, root canals and whatever else were well intact so that I would not have to worry about my teeth while I was abroad. He took the time to check me out thoroughly, and shortly after Joseph and I were off to Japan. Excited does not begin to describe how I felt!

Several months into our stay, I was eating at a restaurant when I realized my bridge was floating in my mouth! "This can't be happening," I thought. My wonderful adventure was suddenly taking a frightening turn. A health challenge while abroad was a nightmare I had hoped to avoid. And this was double trouble! I was not only going to have to deal with a dentist, but I also had to have one who did not speak English! The only consolation was that a Japanese friend, who accompanied me on doctor visits, could serve as my translator.

We made it to the dentist office, but upon arrival it was explained that things were not done the same way in Japan as they were in the USA. I remember thinking, "What does that mean?" Those nightmare images of my youth were slowly creeping back into my mind. I tried to stay calm as I listened to the translation telling me that we were babies in the USA. As if that were not enough to offend my sense of patriotism, he continued his rant. He told me I would not be given medication to relieve any pain that I might experience because he had no prior medical records concerning me. "Is he mad?", I screamed in my head. "No Novocain?" I was suddenly very warm, and it took a moment to realize the grip of fear and panic now commanding my body to *run* and to run *fast* out of his office. As I think back now on an experience best forgotten, I can only wonder how much sadistic pleasure the dentist may have had in seeing the horror engulf my face as my friend was translating. This was fear in its purest form. But my feet didn't move. When my friend and I left the office, I asked her if she knew of another dentist to which she responded, "Oh you are lucky to get him. He's the best." I was in a state of shock. How was I going to endure a much-needed procedure when I was so afraid?

The day of the procedure I was shaking so badly that I imagined I might die, and that's not an exaggeration. To add to my anxiety, I learned that my friend–my translator, the only witness to my torture–would not be able to accompany me. I was on my own. Oddly, despite my current state of fear, I finally understood my husband's apprehension about living in a foreign country where English was not commonly spoken. I wondered if he was as afraid at the prospect of living abroad as I was at that moment.

Returning to the events, years later, of my back surgery, I have come to realize that there is only one thing that many of us actually fear: **DEATH.**

Once we realize that we are alive—and choose to live—we may become afraid of anything that could jeopardize life. I remember lying in the hospital and thinking there is nothing I can change about my situation. It was what it was. I could not wish the situation away nor could I hurry it along. I could only go through it by taking one moment at a time. When I saw my toes move, it was evidence that I was not alone. I was never alone, even during my dental experience in Japan. For years I saw myself as being alone and it perpetuated my many fears. Such fallacy taught me to expect the worse. But the rest I had allowed myself to take in the hospital and in Christ Jesus, was a reminder to me that I was truly never alone. In my weakest state of being, I was made strong and I grew stronger when I realized I was in God's hands.

Before the surgery resulting in the spinal cord injury, I believed that my relationship with God was a good one. I believed in Him. I prayed to Him. I read my Bible, and I even meditated on Him. Nevertheless, I would often find myself caught in a situation where I feared what man might do to me. I remember writing a letter to my parents telling them that I was a very fearful person. I wanted to please everyone so that there would never be any tension with anyone. Although I served God, the fear of death still ran rampant in my mind. I believed the Holy Spirit was telling me that God wanted to use me, but I could not move forward. My fears paralyzed me. Despite there being no basis to imagine the worse would happen, I still believed it would. As a result, I often remained frozen, so traumatized I was not allowing God to use me, all because of fear. Unfortunately, I had read what the Word of God said, but fear kept me from believing it. Many times I have read *1 John 4:18* which tells me perfect love does not embrace fear. How many times have I wondered if I could even consider myself a royal child of the King? And so, I was tormented over and over.

Yet embracing my experience in the hospital finally made the scripture come alive to my innermost being. I laid on my back looking up. I realized that if God had wanted to take me out of this world, He had ample opportunity. Instead, He first restored life into my stilled body. As I observed life in the form of two toes moving, I realized that God was allowing me to witness in slow motion, His grandeur. I dared not miss the wonder of these moment-by-moment acts of God. Tears flowed from my eyes as I realized just how much He loves me. He was keeping me as I was walking through the valley of the shadow of death.

That is exactly what I was to remember: I was not in death but in a shadow. A shadow is not that which is actual. The enemy wants us to focus on the shadows. Vision is obscured in a shadow; you can't see clearly. Fear lurks in the shadows. Fear is not about what actually *is* but what is perceived or threatened. What a liberating concept. Understanding God's immense love for me and knowing I did not have to fear lifted a burden I had carried for a long time. This realization comforted me during my stay in the hospital. I did not lose a night's sleep. In fact, I was eager to sleep to see what the next day would bring. The absence of fear brings an overwhelming flood of love and joy. I could laugh and be the model patient I believed God wanted me to be. I knew I was in the hospital because I needed to get to where God needed me to be. He wanted me to fully understand how He so loves the world and that includes me.

I learn daily to love God with a love that surpasses the love I have for any other. I am no longer afraid of what can happen to me because I know that God will never leave me nor forsake me. Resting in this assurance helps me to understand all is well. He loves me so much and knowing He does makes me adore Him the more. I am excited to be in His presence and to bask in His aura.

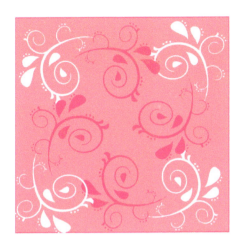

Chapter 7:

RETHINKING PATIENCE

And so, after he had patiently endured, he obtained the promise.
(Hebrews 6:15)

I can remember when Julius was very young, still in a highchair. I was about to serve him dinner. My son loved to eat and after getting settled in his chair, he picked up his fork. He knew exactly what time it was. A moment before placing his meal in front of him, I looked out the window and could see his father walking towards the house coming home from work. I turned back to my son with his fork lifted up by his tiny arms to declare the start of the eating race, "Let's go mom. Bring on the eats!" I looked at him and responded, as though his thoughts were audible, "We have to wait. Daddy's coming." Julius put down his fork and waited. His father arrived and we greeted each other with a kiss. Joseph greeted Julius with a pat on the head. We then moved everything into the dining room and I placed a dinner serving on the table for my husband. How sweet it was for Julius to wait. There was no temper tantrum as one might have anticipated a hungry child could create. Once one was called to the high chair, what would be so important as to hold up the eats? Maybe he knew that we traditionally ate this meal as a family. Maybe he recognized his Daddy was missing. Regardless as to why he responded to my voice so calmly, I fondly remember the patience he demonstrated for someone of his age.

As Julius grew older, there were other situations where he demonstrated the same extraordinary patience. His wait list included the family car we desperately needed, the drum set he asked of Santa Claus for Christmas, a trip to Disney World, and even the house that seemed improbable for us to purchase. To say that he was passionate about these items is an understatement. Julius was politely insistent that something had to be done to get these things. Yet, he never had a temper or acted unseemly because he did not receive what he wanted when he wanted them. When I told him that he had to wait for Santa to make his wish come true or if I said we had to wait on God that was enough. He seemed perfectly content to know that God was working things out for us. I do not mean to imply that he did not remind me of the items on his wish list, but, he never seemed to pout. Somehow, reminding Julius that his request was heard, acknowledged and on the way appeared to be all that he needed to activate an amazing amount of patience.

When I think back on the days Julius saw each request unfold, I can only remember the sense of glee and in some cases amazement that what he had asked for had actually arrived. Julius had wanted the new family car so badly, he asked to buy his dad a toy van for Christmas. The toy came with a card from Julius. In it, Julius told his father that he knew God would bring him a car soon. Soon came two months later. It was a brown passenger van. You would have thought the car was Julius'. He ran to the van smiling from ear to ear as he got in the rear passenger's seat. I can also vividly remember the sound of the scream he made when he saw his drum set under the Christmas tree. It wasn't a piercing sound or like when he falls and hurts himself. It was a sweet sound, almost melodic, hitting notes and decibels that let everyone know he was happy. He even mentioned he did not know how Santa got them in the house without his knowledge. Honestly, I too remain amazed at how Santa did it, but I know it was not easy.

The final two requests were the biggest requests Julius had as a child. They were also the ones that were most costly! They were the ones that brought me and Joseph to our knees! Joseph and I prayed together often so it wasn't the process that was different, it was the request because we didn't have any idea how to make it happen. We didn't have the money and we didn't know how we were going to get it. Our prayer was about making Julius' biggest two dreams come true.

The first request was to go to Disney World. When Julius first asked Santa, Mommy and Daddy even thought Santa would be able to work something out. After many unsuccessful attempts that year, the numbers we needed just didn't mesh with our budget. That Christmas Julius did not get what he most wanted. Yet, his response to the news was almost immeasurable. In fact, if you weren't paying attention, you would have missed his brief display of disappointment; it was rather fleeting. I was more disappointed than he was, yet, in that moment, I watched my child move on. He laughed and smiled and enjoyed unwrapping the gifts that Santa did bring.

I had wanted Julius to have an amazing Disney experience. He was into the Toy Story characters, with Buzz Light Year and Woody being his favorites. He had the toys and of course he could almost recite the movie verbatim. I wanted him to be in the hotel where the characters would be roaming around. I also could just imagine the conversations Julius would have with them. Yes, I wanted Julius to have a full-blown Disney experience. What was I thinking? The cost of such a vacation was indeed out of our reach especially during the Christmas season. Joseph suggested we continue planning for the trip and that I tone down the extravagant way I was hoping to present Disney World to Julius. Eventually, things worked out. I had to remember that our thoughts are not always God's thoughts, and our ways are not His ways. Sometimes our timing is not even God's timing. We must remember to ask Him when and how to do what we want. Lots of hardship can be saved if we consider Him in all our ways.

On the day of the trip, Julius woke up and got dressed as though it were any other day in third grade. He did not know we were headed to the airport. It was a day I will never forget. We already had everything packed and then the moment came. All the planning, secrets, whispering and joy was for this moment. We told him this would not be an ordinary day and that we were not going to follow our usual routine. While he stared at us with puzzled eyes, we screamed, "We're going to Disney World!" Julius jumped and danced all around the living room in jubilee. The joy I felt recording my mind video has never left me and I suspect it never will.

When Julius was eleven, I spent the summer looking for what he called, "our new house." Second to having "our new house" was the excitement of taking the yellow school bus. Somehow in his early school years, Julius internalized that his friends that took the school bus were more advantaged than he was. In my mind, it was debatable because Julius was driven to school. I would argue that he was in a better position, but the mind of a child is simply not always understandable. He may have been envious because the school bus children were dismissed from school earlier and he had to stay at school longer. Anyway, signing him up for bus transportation was merely our secret parental way to transition him to get ready to take the bus from our new home.

That September we closed on the house, but it wasn't until the end of September that the final transition took place. I suggested to Joseph that we should surprise Julius. Joseph would pick Julius up from school and bring him to our new home. I was waiting there with the video camera in hand to film Julius' reaction to another one of his answered prayer requests. Needless to say, the joy he expressed was indescribable although I can replay the event in my mind over and over. I taped him going from room to room. I saw him stop. Unprompted, he bowed his head and told God "thank you." I don't know how I kept my composure.

Julius waited a long time for some of his prayer requests. He waited patiently and with an unwavering determination that they would be answered. What is it that allows us to demonstrate such patience? Why do we have patience in some circumstances but not in others? I found my answer in Julius. In each situation, he demonstrated a sense of gratefulness and trust in his parents and ultimately in God. He waited for what he wanted, and when it arrived, he was grateful. He appeared to blindly trust that what he had asked for would come true. He trusted in what he believed to be true–Santa, his parents, and God. He had an established relationship with each of them. All the while he was building trust in God who knows just how to make everything happen to make our hearts glad.

When I started this writing journey, Julius had enrolled in the community college. It had been over a year since the onset of my affliction. Our family income had been compromised. I remember thinking we would really have to trust God to help us get him through college. Once again God came to our rescue. Our first break came when the state decided to pay tuition for students attending state schools. Julius decided on his own to attend the community college and commute from home. What a blessing!

Julius was ready to transfer to complete his bachelor's degree before we knew it. There was an announcement in which he informed us that he only wanted to attend one college at the university where we lived. He had no desire to apply anywhere else. There was a silent war between us as I had to insist that he apply to some of the state schools or any of the other schools across the nation. As the acceptance and award letters came in, we were thrilled. Julius actually had choices. Still Julius waited for that *one* award letter. Finally, the school of his choice was really the school of his choice! He was not only accepted but the award letter superseded what we had ever anticipated. He was awarded enough to attend the school he wanted including its summer session. Once again, I saw him respond with an attitude of gratefulness so humbling it brought tears to my eyes.

I believe, a spirit of gratefulness is what moves the heart of God. He is constantly looking for us to say, "Thank you." Do you remember the biblical story of the ten lepers that Jesus healed? Jesus told them to go and show themselves to the priest, and they did. Only one returned to thank him and Jesus wondered aloud where the other nine were (Luke 17: 11-19). Throughout my pink experience, I have tried through every blessing, pain, disappointment, victory and even the unknown to be the one to return and tell God, "Thank You."

Thank you. Two words, three or more if you call Him by name. Telling God thank you has made my situation more bearable because I am reminded that things could always be worse. Practicing gratitude reminded me that there was still good in the world and victories coming my way. When I woke up unable to move my legs, I was able to say, "Thank you" because I still had my faculties. I could still do some things for myself, and I was still assured that God had not left me. When God told me that I would have my ministry after the surgery, that alone was something for which to be grateful.

In my church organization, a woman who is licensed to work in ministry is called a missionary. I was called to serve as a missionary six years prior to my fall. I have fed the poor, visited the sick, prayed intercessory prayers, taught bible classes and even prepared messages to encourage people to accept Christ as their Lord and Savior. Some would say I fulfilled the duties customary to a missionary's calling. Yet, I did not know my true mission. I always felt there was a higher purpose for my calling. I often inquired of the Lord and I always received the same answer: "Wait."

Over the years, like my son, I have received more from God than I could ever have imagined. His grace has taken me to several countries, allowed me to excel in my work, and blessed me with Joseph and Julius and a happy home. I was anxious to have a family. I was nearing thirty and it seemed as though I would never walk down the aisle, but I waited patiently because I knew that I only wanted what God wanted for me. I remember telling the Lord that if He wanted me to remain single, I was contented because He had been so good to me. I even considered what I would do as a single woman. Perhaps I would have the opportunity to go all over the world to see the places my God had created.

Well, as you know, I did get married, but Julius did not come right away. I was thankful that I could honestly be happy without anything in my quiver because God had been so good to me. After five years of marriage, I was content that if it was the will of God to be childless, no problem. Shortly after, I discovered a child was on the way, and I was thankful. I suppose what I want to convey is that waiting can be tough. It can be disappointing. It can even be frustrating. There were periods of time when waiting even made me think things were never going to work out. However, through all the waiting, I remained happy in the Lord. I was trusting and believing in Him.

Waiting is a big part of how I continue to heal from my affliction. I have learned to be patient in so many ways, with myself, with the healing process, and with how the body restores itself. I had to learn to be patient about the upkeep of my home. It now takes great effort for it to be as tidy as I would like it to be. I have learned to pace myself and thank God for what He allows me to accomplish day by day. I have learned to be patient with others in their kindness to meet my needs. Care takers want to help, make you comfortable and keep you from overtaxing yourself. But accepting their help was sometimes a challenge, and I wanted to say, "Just let me do it, I'm okay." But often, receiving assistance is the godly thing to do. Allowing others to accommodate my needs, to go to appointments or just walking with me to get a breath of fresh air, demonstrates God's love. I am grateful for every act of kindness.

In rethinking patience, I conclude that it is the state of contentment that allows one to accept the will of God for whatever we ask. That state of contentment leads one to say thank you knowing that whatever God wants you to have, you will have only in His time, not yours. Contentment opens the door for exploring in the meantime. In the meantime, how will you react to the circumstance, to the prayer request, to waiting? Will you have a temper tantrum or be able to exhibit total calm? Will you have thoughts of indignation or be able to totally trust God? Will you have a negative attitude or an attitude of utmost gratitude?

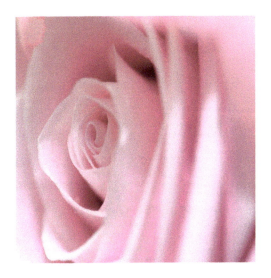

Chapter 8:

RETHINKING LONELINESS

Lo I am with you always, even unto the end of the world. Amen.
(Matthew 28:20b)

I love music, particularly good gospel music. It always makes me feel as though I am never alone. One of the most enduring things about music is that technology allows it to go everywhere. As a gospel music lover, I took my cassette tapes and Walkman wherever I went. When I was seventeen, I took them to Barcelona, Spain as a high school senior. The music culture did not share in my appreciation of Black gospel music. The Internet, YouTube and other recent day modes of music indulgence were not to be found. I think I would have felt very alone had I not had the foresight to pack cassette tapes and my Walkman. I was part of a program dedicated to immersing junior and senior high students in the Spanish language and culture.

I lived with a Spanish speaking family and was treated as a member. Actually, I lived with two families; the first would often speak Catalan, a language of the Basque ethnicity, and the other would speak primarily Castilian Spanish, most similar to the language learned in school textbooks. In the Basque family, Mama would sometimes translate the Catalan to Castilian Spanish so I would have some idea of what was being said. I learned a few expressions, my favorite being: *"He tingut prou!"* (I've had enough!) Mama would say this quite often as her daughters were always trying her patience in some manner. She had five daughters: three were married, one was engaged and the youngest was always paired with me.

Every Sunday the family came together with their spouses and her one and only grandson to feast and rattle off in Catalan. Those were difficult days. A feeling of loneliness in the midst of the continuous chatter was sometimes more than I could bare. I think I longed most for my family at those dinners. While I would marvel at how quickly they spoke, they reminded me of family gatherings at my grandmother's house with aunts, uncles and cousins floating in and out. I never felt alone at grandma's house. The relationship between each of my relatives was always one of pride and belonging. I was my grandparents' granddaughter, my aunts' and uncles' niece, my cousins' cousin my parents' daughter, my brother's older younger sister and my sister's older sister. I was well defined and proudly took my place in the midst of them all. Good relationships were expected of me by my parents. Yet as much as I appreciated my Catalan family, there was always a sense of isolation when I was in their presence. Those were days when my Walkman was of greatest comfort. I would go in my room and let the music assist me to fall asleep.

Perhaps my loneliness was due to the language barrier. During the time I was in Spain, there were no wonders of social media as there are today. Snail mail coupled with outrageous international phone call prices kept me feeling the distance and separation from my family. I actually left the family because I believed I was not grasping the language and the isolation I felt at the time seemed unbearable. Ultimately, I was transferred to another home, with a family that spent a lot of time talking to me. The father was an editor of one of the newspapers and the mother was a homemaker with two little girls I looked forward to seeing each day. They welcomed my presence on their Sunday family outings, and I do believe my language ability greatly improved due to my familiarity with Castilian and their intentional efforts to converse with me. I did not feel so much as an outsider and so the loneliness was not as prevalent as it had been before. In this instance, loneliness was lessened by a sense of verbal inclusion.

Another time, I was living in Costa Rica with a family where the lady of the house spoke English well. She was closer to me in age and so we acted more as sisters. I would often be included in family gatherings. One day I was invited to attend a wedding reception for one of the family members. There again, the wedding guests reminded me of my family–they laughed and enjoyed the celebration of two large clans coming together as one. As I observed the festivities, I noticed a sparkle coming from an ice sculpture. As I stood there wondering what was causing the twinkle, a little girl came and gave me a ribbon with a pin that if the sun hit it just so, it sparkled. I do not know what made her think to give me the ribbon, but it was a moment I always remember as one which God hears and knows my thoughts afar off. More importantly, I am never alone because He is always tangibly present.

I can think of a number of times when I have been physically alone but have not felt a twinge of loneliness. At other times I am lonely. Generally, loneliness is defined as the absence of others. I think it goes deeper than this. In my experiences abroad, there were other people around me. When these people tried to reach out to me, if I responded to their friendliness, the loneliness left. When I could not connect, the feeling of loneliness persisted. This observation has led me to rethink, "what is loneliness?" It is more than physical isolation because it has mental and emotional components. In order for physical isolation not to become a state of loneliness, one has to be comfortable being with oneself. When the company of others is needed to validate our existence, then being alone is an existential crisis.

When one is not in the presence of others, the only way to avoid the concept of loneliness is to acknowledge the company of being with oneself. Sickness and affliction tend to make one believe the sickness is only about the individual in the hospital or laying at home in the bed. How important it is to be satisfied with one's own being in the fight for wellness. The degree of self-confidence and worth determines the degree of success. When one is not mentally connected with others nor oneself, deterioration occurs. Therefore, patients must value the person they are. They have to be able to enjoy their own company.

The decision to stay in Rochester to recover after surgery was primarily mine. I was helpless in so many ways and I felt as though the initial days of recovery had yielded great progress. I felt as though I would receive the best care if I did not interrupt the recovery process by trying to return to Syracuse. Although Joseph surmised that this would mean a longer separation, he agreed. I can still see his conflicted look of support and despair when he left me behind and headed back home. The separation Joseph and I experienced was not our first. As a school teacher, I had the same long vacations as Julius. School would end and it was a matter of a few days before we were packed and hitting the road out of town. We always said our prayer of separation. I'd kiss Joseph good-bye, grab Julius and away we would go to visit family and friends and at least to smell the ocean. I'd tell myself we were also giving Joseph a vacation from us; he would have the house completely to himself without any interruption to whatever he was doing. We just believed God would bring us together again and He always did. But the stay in the hospital was different. It was a separation we had not planned. When separation is unexpected, it can be overwhelming.

From the start of my ordeal, I promised myself that I was going to do whatever was necessary to walk again. As I have already stated, during my time on the acute therapy ward, many people complained that they wanted to go home, often crying about how much they missed their home and family. I cannot say that I did not miss Joseph or Julius. I can say that I did not have a feeling of loneliness. My hospital recovery required me to focus on two tasks: 1) walking out of the hospital, and 2) operating in the mission God had given me. In order to walk out of the hospital, I had to focus on every physical exercise I was told to perform. My day as an acute patient included two hours of physical and occupational therapy as well as a social therapy session. To get ready for the active day, I would wake up about 6:00 a.m. I wanted time for my morning prayer, and to watch my favorite televangelists. I loved to follow the messages given to Joyce Myers, T.D. Jakes, David Jerimiah, Charles Stanley and Creflo Dollar. Some televangelists I watched were new to me. I particularly appreciated being introduced to the teachings of Robert Morris, Jimmy Evans, Kerry Shook and Steven Furtick.

I do not remember whether or not there was a radio in my room. At home I would awaken to the radio and hear a teaching program and songs of praise before I got out of bed. But in the acute ward I substituted television ministries for the radio programs I used to rely on. I would awaken to a good gospel message every morning. So many people lived through their cell phones and had to begin their day cruising social media. I have to admit, I had not (and still have not) caught up to the present in the world of personal technology. It was one day after having social therapy that I realized there was a computer in the room that was available for my use. I was so happy because the music I could only remember in my head I could now search for and play into the atmosphere. I could close the door to the room and sing to my heart's content. I only remember being asked to vacate the room once for another patient. Sometimes others would join me in conversation.

After my devotional time in the morning, I got ready for therapy. For many other patients this was a time of dread, but I actually looked forward to it. For me it meant I was getting closer to going home. It meant that I was getting better. I found joy in striving to accomplish more than the day before. Therapy for me was watching God perform daily miracles. I know not everyone felt this way. Having a love for people, it was also my privilege to hear the hearts of others as they shared their struggles with me.

Many wanted, but were unable, to have a positive outlook on their experience. What do you say to a 25-year-old mother who is recovering from a stray bullet that paralyzed her and separated her from her two little boys? How do you encourage a woman who chose to be proactive with her health, but her decisions resulted in leg amputation? When a man questions God for not taking his life instead of having him live with what he sees is an unbearably diminished body, what words of comfort can be offered? Our shared therapy sessions were my opportunities to try to cheer them all on. It was my time to listen, empathize and support those who needed a little consolation or encouragement. It was the time to push myself and them through the process of mental and physical healing, the process of believing the impossible was possible and the gradual understanding that if God had brought us this far, He was not about to leave us alone now.

As you can see my desire to recover was in sync with doing God's will. It seemed all I had to do was find a way to help someone else and I would also be helping myself. Listening to others does not leave much time to dwell on personal thoughts of discomfort and allows the new norm to be tolerated while maintaining a positive attitude to improve. I sincerely listened to what mattered to others; what they had been through; their fears. Listening made me realize how grateful I am that my situation was not worse.

Sometimes the afternoon workouts were quieter as not many people were scheduled for a session. This was when I would hear about the lives of the therapists. They were all younger than me and very vibrant. They called themselves the A-Team not just because their names all began with the letter "A" but because they saw themselves as the 1980s television A-Team: no case was too hard for them to pull through. My A-team was phenomenal! When I was teaching, I remember hearing that a student will work harder for a teacher they liked. I think it's true. I liked the A-team and I know I worked harder. I wanted to match their level of enthusiasm and commitment to my recovery with my efforts in therapy. With my A-team, I was not alone, I had at least three cheerleaders every day to keep me going strong.

Upon returning to my room, I had time for a nap before the evening dinner cart would appear. I hate to admit it, but I was always delighted to see my meal arrive. I'd watch a little television and then eagerly awaited my faithful callers: Mom, my sister Lysa, and Joseph. I did not realize the extent to which my mother felt she needed to be with me (or I needed to be with her) until I saw her for the first time about a year later after my operation. I suppose I should have felt lonely for her, but I was able to talk with her every night as I usually did when I was home. I am sure that satiated my desire to see her.

When I first got to the hospital, I did not have a cellphone. Once Mom was able to call me directly through the hospital line, her voice was the medicine a daughter needed. We always had something to laugh about. I particularly appreciated the more intimate talks where we could share, especially those matters of the body that a lady would never discuss in public. My body was changing, evolving and I was fortunate to have Mom so that she could help me figure out what was going on. Nevertheless, with all the telephone conversations, I did not realize how necessary it was for her to see me with her eyes and confirm that all was progressing well. As much as I assured her that I was all right, nothing made any sense to her until I was physically in her presence.

When we finally were together, she shared the pain she felt not being able to be with me. She felt alienated from her child. My father also shared, in his fatherly way, his sense of sadness in the inability to come see what affliction had beset his child. Separation from my parents was not new to me. Since the age of fifteen there was always a reason that we were not together. They afforded me so many wonderful opportunities because they were willing to let me go to boarding school, travel abroad to Spain, Costa Rica and Japan, and move away to live with my husband. Hearing their comments was hard and brought tears to my eyes. I had missed them too, and the moments reunited with them brought a revelation: I was lonely without them. Nevertheless, God is amazing in that all the experiences I have had without my parents made it possible to move forward in my pink journey. He gave me to focus more on the mission of encouraging others than on my personal needs. I'm so glad He did!

During my stay, it was perhaps most difficult to wrestle with knowing my son Julius was growing up without me. I wondered whether our separation would cause him to act out in some unpredictable way. Was he strong enough to be alone? Had he been prepared for such a time as this? Was he okay being on his own while his father came to visit me in Rochester? How did he feel knowing he only had fleeting glimpses of his father, who despite trying to raise his son appeared to have had three other priorities: working, going to the hospital and getting rest? I wondered whether or not

Julius was confiding in someone. Who was he turning to so he could express whatever was on his mind during this time of family crisis? Was he bearing this family burden alone?

Thinking of Julius' plight, I must also think of my husband, my best friend for life. While I cannot possibly know what was passing through his mind, I can say that sometimes it is impossible to know just how lonely one can be when they're without their better half. Joseph had no words for the experience we went through. He had already said he hoped to talk about it when it is over. Even as I write, it is not over. I still have issues walking and complications, primarily neurological concerns, that have not been rectified. The more I say I have been blessed through the ordeal, the more Joseph looks at me as if to say, "Are you nuts? Have you no idea how horrible things have been for me? Am I the only one who realizes what an awfully lonely experience this has been without you by my side? Do you realize how difficult it was for a me to drive alone to and from Rochester? Do you know how empty and lonely the house is without you? And worse of all, do you realize how difficult it was knowing I was too tired to be with you every night and had to suffice with just a phone call?"

And let's not forget my sister, my closest friend. She is the person who I learned to love for who she is. I can only imagine what it is like to have three of your immediate family members (mother, father and sister) in the hospital at the same time, all at a distance while being careful not to trigger your own health issues. Knowing my sister, I know it was challenging for her – especially verbally. She is an open person and "puts it all out there," so, I am sure she was being especially careful with what she said. She didn't want to trigger any negative energy. But for a good while, she lost her shopping-spree partner, her "girl's night out" buddy, her laugh out loud tickler. So, for a period of time, stretched far beyond what she would have wished, I know she was feeling alone. We're just that connected.

My brother John Darryl stayed with me in spirit during my hospital stay. As my big brother, he has always looked out for a me even though we are separated by great distance. He has always been on his post of making sure I was all right by calling frequently. Mom believes it's because we shared the cradle and were always close. I grew up knowing and believing he was my forever hero. I felt most contented hearing the voice of each one of my immediate family. These were the ones I believe not only loved me but were praying continually for me. They were my praying family A-team. Many people did not know the affliction that had befallen me, but when they heard, God used their calls and prayers to keep me from being lonely.

The nurses and aids on my ward considered me a good patient because I would try to be as cheerful as possible. I wanted them to know if no one else in their care appreciated them, I did. I greeted them each day with a warm "good morning" and was glad to tell them I had rested well the night before. Most of the time I did. I can only remember one roommate, an elderly woman who wanted to get out of bed and would try to take off the restraints that had to be put on her to prevent her from walking out of bed. She had tried all night to get out of bed. They say medication can have different effects on a person especially through the dosage regulation period. That night I prayed for her even though I did not know if she understood what was happening. I guess I did not want her to feel alone.

In the morning I learned from her daughter that she was a Christian and would soon turn ninety years young. I never would have guessed her age. She was well preserved. After that night, her family became my "family." Even her grandchildren would come and talk with me when they came to visit. One day when I returned from therapy, there was a wonderful book about phenomenal women of the Bible on my bed. One of the daughters found the book in the supermarket. She said she thought of me immediately.

It was her way to say thank you for not letting her mother be alone during the night. I still feel like I am holding a treasure when I read it.

I may never understand the depth of the physical, mental and emotional separation each of my family members experienced. I am aware that my affliction has made us all have to adjust to a new normal. God covered my family and me from feeling the depth of loneliness and separation in a difficult hour. I believe God heard every detail of my prayers as I asked Him to take care of my family and me during our unexpected separation. Just like the people in my therapy sessions, there was a process to go through that made us endure loneliness and separation. I believe God allowed me to be a cheerleader for each of my family members and friends. In truth, we were never completely alone.

No, I was never alone.

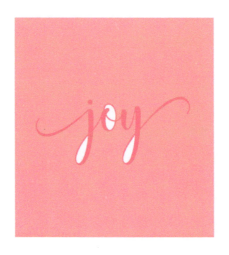

Chapter 9:

RETHINKING PINK AGAIN

"Let us hear the conclusion of the whole matter: Fear God, and keep his commandments: for this is the whole duty of man."
                              (Ecclesiastes 12:13)

In my church, Mother's Day has always been well celebrated by women dressing up and sporting the latest fashion. For some women it would mean not only a new dress but all the accessories too. The finery includes shoes, hat, pocketbook and gloves, as well as the appropriate adorning jewelry, to match the dress or suit and to become the most eye-catching outfit. My first Mother's Day, I was so elated to be a mother that I wanted to take part in the church hoopla. I dressed in the soft pink dress coat I found and dressed my young son in his powder blue outfit. I found myself eagerly looking forward to the picture that would capture the moment. (Yes, I know exactly where it is!) When Mother's Day was over, I wore the dress from time to time until I had to retire it. I did not have another pink dress for some time.

Second Sunday in my local church is Women's Day. In the spirit of unity, women are asked to wear white. We have changed our dress code over the years so that now the women wear whatever the facilitators for the month suggest. Once after the color chosen was pink, someone heard me say I didn't like pink. She said, "You don't like pink and yet you wear that beautiful pink dress?" I do have a really beautiful pink dress. It is pink: not pastel pink, not hot pink, not rose, not fuchsia. It is the only pink dress I own. My parents gave it to me for my birthday one year. I like the style and the material, and I like the way I wear the dress. It makes me feel like a beautiful lady when I wear it. Unfortunately, I can no longer fit the dress, but it still hangs in my closet in anticipation of the day I am focused enough to "battle the bulge" and return to my former dress size. As I think of the two pink dresses that made me feel so special, I am rethinking my personal pink perspective. In my recollection of the times when the color pink was part of a special moment in my life, I have to consider the power of the color.

To my carnal eye, pink was sickness and weakness. Perhaps it even represented a concept of fear within me I was not willing to face. While I was in the hospital, I believe the Spirit of God spoke to my heart to write my testimony which has filled these pages. In reminiscent moments, I realize I have had an amazing spiritual journey in which I have had daily laughter instead of tears, extended patience in place of frustration, and unending love rather than bitterness.

Resting in the Lord has proven to be more beneficial than natural rest. It brought me sweet sleep rather than the insomnia brought on by excessive worry. Spiritual rest encourages me to get up and embrace the dawning of the new day with anticipation. I sincerely believe that today will be better than yesterday, even if I encounter a setback of some sort. Spiritual rest prevented me from asking "why is this happening to me?" and helped me realize God was *using* me to help everyone around me. It was about acknowledging the faithfulness of the Almighty God and respecting His sovereignty!

Yes, resting in God allows us to look all around and notice every created being in such a miniscule space in the world. Rest helps us to hear the neighbor that cries out and compels us to intercede. It helps us discern the individuality and uniqueness of everyone we meet. There are so many people that contribute to making our world what we think it is. It requires us to step back and look at each person and ask, "Did I pray for every individual and ask God in His omniscient way to take care of their needs so that in turn my needs are also met?" "Am I indeed aware of my community and all that it entails?" "Have I taken time to appreciate everyone and everything for the role they play in my life?" "Have I thanked God for His orchestration of the details, since everything is working out for my good?

Spiritual rest also helped me to see a group of people I may not have fully noticed before. I have visited the sick and afflicted in the hospital and even in their home. I have dropped in when I had penciled in 30 minutes only to discover that more time was required of me, and I have made that sacrifice. I have prayed for those who have had to have an operation or were confronting a life-threatening disease and did not know how to get up and move forward. But what have I actually given to the disabled, the blind, the lame, the deaf or dumb? How desirous I have become to spend time in their presence in an effort to comfort and encourage them, until they can see for themselves the love of God.

I now have an intimate understanding of the scripture which says those who are well need no physician. I so want to be able to impart the understanding that the fear of disability is so often coupled with the spirit of fear. That fear for many is social rejection. As social beings, no one wants to be alone or to be a burden to another. Either feeling can result in depression, which if not addressed can bring on the delusion that death is better than living. This is exactly why I believe I was given the task to first rest and listen to how much I was loved by God. God is love and perfect love casts out fear. I know that my pink journey could have been one of the gloomiest experiences of my life. Had I not had the love of God coursing through my being, I wouldn't have been able to glorify God or to sing praises unto Him. Resting in God gave me the opportunity to clear my mind, concentrate on the love of God, and accordingly receive His blessings day by day.

With no fear in my mind or heart, God was able to use my physical body as an illustration of how He works through abnormal circumstances to produce amazing experiences. Frankly, I would have also been very impatient with myself and with those around me. But so often I hear myself coaching my body to "take it easy" and to "take your time." I can laugh when it sometimes seems to take so long to get dressed that, about the time I do, it is almost time to change for bed. I can chuckle to myself when someone holding open a door for me says, "Take your time," as if I could possibly move faster. I am learning to be patient with myself as well as with others. Although I find that there are times when I still want healing to happen immediately, there has been great strength in my affliction. That is when I talk to the Lord and ask for Him to calm my spirit. I do not wish to be a spoiled Christian brat. I want to be a devoted child of God because He has truly been devoted to me.

All along my journey, I have had to admit, God has never left me alone. From the time I first laid on the floor in agony, to the doctor's prognosis, to the recovery room, through acute therapy and home healing, I have never been alone. God promised me He would never leave me nor forsake me. I have not found one of His promises unkept. Does this mean I am back to full range of motion? WOW, wouldn't that be the great storybook ending!

So, let's take a look at where I am now. Physically, I am finding more time to exercise daily. For the few years after surgery, I made the mistake of staying in the house during the very cold winters. I wanted to stay curled up in my chair, blanket on top, ready for cozy winter naps. I strongly recommend, if it is at all possible, move the body every hour on the hour and drink water. Incontinence is still of great concern and is common among SCI patients. Nevertheless, trips to the bathroom definitely keep one moving.

I'm not as active as I want to be, but I stay in therapy, and I have found some good classes at a nearby gym to strengthen my balance and work my core muscles. It's always intriguing to see which muscles want to work one day but not another. My goal is to make it outside at least 3-4 times a week in winter. Classes have also increased my social development. Since starting my classes, the turnover rate of new people coupled with class time changes gives me opportunity to not only share my story but to hear the stories of others. And guess what? We can really root for one another. But what I do more than anything is pray. I know that I can be an intercessor for the people with more aches and pains than one might want to hear about.

As we stretch and move, I have learned to talk to God on behalf of those who need Jehovah Raffa – God Our Healer. And I believe the prayers work not just because of me but because there are others in the class that are praying also. At the beginning of class, I have heard someone say how bad they felt but after the workout the pain was gone or subsided. I can concur. But I can also do a little too much and then have to decide whether or not I should endure the pain or fight the grogginess that comes with quicker working muscle relaxers. Rarely do I choose the medication. I simply take time to rest and remind myself to be patient.

In rethinking pink, I now have several pink items in my wardrobe. I even have a pink toothbrush. That's a major development showing how I have changed! I have several pink journals and who knows how else I will expand my pink collection. I have not yet thought about painting a room in my house pink; nevertheless, I have watched home decorating shows and thought, "Oh I see how pink could work." And although I cannot yet imagine wanting a pink car, I want to drive my own car so badly that I could consent to driving a pink one. That would really be an example of rethinking pink.

Rethinking pink simply means taking time to seek out what God is perfecting in you through the dark times in your life. From a natural perspective, something is happening to me that I may not necessarily like. I may feel trapped, cornered, frustrated, confused, isolated or just ready to give up and die. While the circumstances may indeed be dark, there are still footsteps along the path that are not my own. Indeed, they are the footsteps that are leading me through the valley of the shadow of death and so I do not have to fear. They are the footsteps that encourage me to go on along the path because the way has already been paved. I asked the Lord, "Will I be afflicted for the rest of my life?" I believe He answered, "No." I smiled and said, "Lord, I know I must be specific when I ask you a question so will I be able to enjoy a restored range of motion, complete healing, for a long period of time on this side of life?" I believe He said, "Yes."

CPSIA information can be obtained
at www.ICGtesting.com
Printed in the USA
BVHW091919221022
650018BV00003B/18